ASTHMA

THE MEDICAL PERSPECTIVES SERIES

Advisors:

Andrew P. Read *Department of Medical Genetics, University of Manchester, Manchester, U.K.*

Terence Brown *Department of Biochemistry and Applied Molecular Biology, UMIST, Manchester, U.K.*

Michael Kerr *Department of Pathology, Ninewells Hospital and Medical School, Dundee, U.K.*

Robin Winter *Institute of Child Health, London, U.K.*

Oncogenes and Tumor Suppressor Genes

Cytokines

The Human Genome

Autoimmunity

Genetic Engineering

Asthma

Molecular Virology (due 1994)

ASTHMA

A.J. Wardlaw
Department of Respiratory Medicine, University of Leicester Medical School and Glenfield General Hospital, Groby Road, Leicester LE3 9QP, U.K.

βIOS
SCIENTIFIC
PUBLISHERS

First published in the United Kingdom 1993 by
BIOS Scientific Publishers Limited,
St Thomas House, Becket Street, Oxford OX1 1SJ.

A CIP catalogue record for this book is available from the British Library.

ISBN 1 872748 26 0

To Catherine

Typeset by Marksbury Typesetting Ltd, Midsomer Norton, Bath, U.K.
Printed by Information Press Ltd, Oxford, U.K.

Preface

Asthma affects about 5% of the population of the industrialized nations and there is evidence to suggest that it is increasing in both prevalence and severity. While in many people asthma is readily controlled with available medication, it remains a disease which causes considerable ill health and up to 2000 deaths a year in the UK. Over the last decade there has been a major research effort into the causes of asthma which has transformed our understanding of the disease. Progress has been aided by spectacular advances in the fields of cell and molecular biology, which have unravelled the basis of the immune response and the nature of the inflammatory process. However, as a result, I believe there is an ever widening gap between the specialist, well versed in the finer points of asthma lore, and the student, clinician, health care worker or scientist new to the area, for whom many of the principles involved are foreign and the endless list of mediators and receptors extremely confusing.

A number of excellent and very comprehensive books on asthma are available. They are recommended for further reading at the end of Chapter 1. This book is intended to fill a different need. It is written for the non-asthma specialist in order to provide a general overview of both the clinical features of asthma and the basic mechanisms involved in its pathogenesis. In particular, the book focuses on the way in which recent advances in cell and molecular biology have contributed to our understanding of asthma pathogenesis and the direction which future research and therapies are likely to take. It is intended to be accessible to readers with a limited understanding of immunology and cell biology in order to intepret the very latest advances in our knowledge of this fascinating disease.

A.J. Wardlaw

Acknowledgements

I would like to thank Dr John Cookson and Professor Keith Whaley for their helpful comments, and Stephanie Lloyd for secretarial assistance.

Contents

Abbreviations

ABPA	allergic bronchopulmonary aspergillosis
ACTH	adrenocorticotrophic hormone
APC	antigen-presenting cell
ASA	aspirin sensitive asthma
ATP	adenosine triphosphate
BAL	bronchoalveolar lavage
BALT	bronchial associated lymphoid tissue
BHR	bronchial hyperresponsiveness
BTS	British Thoracic Society
CAO	chronic airflow obstruction
CD	cluster of differentiation
CF	cystic fibrosis
CN-PDE	cyclic nucleotide phosphodiesterase
COAD	chronic obstructive airways disease
COLD	chronic obstructive lung disease
COPD	chronic obstructive pulmonary disease
CRF	corticotrophin-releasing factor
CsA	cyclosporine
CSF	colony-stimulating factor
CXR	chest X-ray
DAG	diacylglycerol
DCG	dense core granulated epithelial cell
DSCG	disodium cromoglycate
EAE	experimental autoimmune encephalitis
ECF-a	eosinophil chemotactic factor of anaphylaxis
ECP	eosinophil cationic protein
EDN	eosinophil derived neurotoxin
EGF	epithelial growth factor
EIA	exercise-induced asthma
EPO	eosinophil peroxidase

Fab	fragment antigen binding
FB	fibrinogen
Fc	fragment crystallizable
FEV_1	forced expiratory volume in one second
FGF	fibroblast growth factor
FKBP	FK-binding protein
FLAP	5-lipoxygenase-activating protein
f-MLP	formyl-methionine, leucine, phenylalanine
FN	fibronectin
FOB	fiber-optic bronchoscopy
FVC	forced vital capacity
GC	glucocorticoid
Glycam	glycosylated cell adhesion molecule
GM-CSF	granulocyte–macrophage colony-stimulating factor
GP	general practitioner
GR	glucocorticoid receptor
GRE	glucocorticoid-responsive element
HDM	house dust mite
HETE	hydroxyeicosatetraenoic acid
HLA	human leukocyte antigen
HSP	heat shock protein
ICAM	intercellular adhesion molecule
IDDM	insulin-dependent diabetes mellitus
IFN-γ	gamma-interferon
Ig	immunoglobulin
IL	interleukin
IP_3	inositol triphosphate
KCO	potassium channel opener
LAD	leukocyte adhesion deficiency disease
LFA-1	lymphocyte function antigen-1
LN	laminin
LT	leukotriene
MAB	monoclonal antibody
Mac-1	macrophage antigen-1
MBP	major basic protein
MCP-1	monocyte chemotactic protein 1
MGSF	melanoma growth-stimulating factor
MHC	major histocompatibility complex
MIP	macrophage inflammatory protein
NANC	non-adrenergic, non-cholinergic
NHLI	National Heart and Lung Institute
NK	natural killer
NSAID	non-steroidal anti-inflammatory drug
PAF	platelet-activating factor
Pc20	provocational concentration causing a 20% fall in FEV_1
PCA	passive cutaneous anaphylaxis

PDE	phosphodiesterase
PF/PEF/	peak flow/peak expiratory flow/
PEFR	peak expiratory flow rate
PG	prostaglandin
PI	phosphatidylinositol
PPIase	proline isomerase
RAST	radioallergoadsorbent test
RB	respiratory bronchiole
RSV	respiratory syncytial virus
SLE	systemic lupus erythematosis
sLex	sialyl Lewis X
SRS-A	slow-reacting substance of anaphylaxis
TB	terminal bronchiole
β-TG	β-thyroglobulin
TGF	transforming growth factor
TNF	tumor necrosis factor
Tx	thromboxane
URTI	upper respiratory tract infections
VCAM	vascular cell adhesion molecule
VIP	vasoactive intestinal peptide
VN	vitronectin

Chapter 1

Clinical aspects of asthma

1.1 What is asthma?

1.1.1 Introduction

Asthma is a common disease of considerable antiquity. It was described by Hippocrates in the fourth century BC and its name derives from the Greek word for panting. Famous sufferers include Marcel Proust, who almost died from a severe attack of asthma at the age of 9, and Samuel Johnson.

The cause of asthma is unknown. Family studies, which are discussed in more detail in Chapter 6, have concluded that there is a genetic component to the disease, but the mode of inheritance is unclear. Support for a genetic component is provided by the high prevalence of asthma in some isolated, in-bred communities, such as in Tristan da Cunha, where

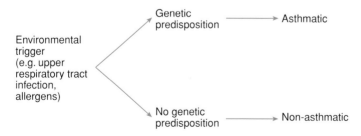

Figure 1.1: Pathogenesis of asthma. Asthma is thought to develop when a genetically susceptible individual is exposed to an environmental stimulus such as an allergen or a viral infection which can trigger an inflammatory reaction in the airways.

1

70% of the population was described as having asthma in the 1940s, as well as differences in prevalence between different racial groups in the same population, as in Singapore and Malaysia, where asthma is less common in the Chinese than in the Indians and Malays. The evidence points to asthma being a disease in which a genetic predisposition to the asthmatic diathesis is expressed only when the at-risk individual comes into contact with an environmental trigger (*Figure 1.1*). It is highly likely that more than one gene controls the predisposition to develop asthma (i.e. it is a multigene disease). The clinical presentation of asthma is very variable, and this has led to the suggestion that it is not one but several diseases, which appear similar because the lung can react only in a limited number of ways to an insult. For example, asthma associated with exposure to substances at work (occupational asthma) may have a different

Table 1.1: Asthma triggers

Group	Examples	Comment
(a) Specific triggers		
Allergens	Grass pollen	'Extrinsic asthmatics'
	House dust mite	
	Cat fur	
Viral infections	Rhinovirus	Upper respiratory tract infections (URTI) are
	Respiratory syncytial virus	one of the commonest triggers, although the virus involved is often not identified
Occupational agent	Acid anhydrides	Colophony in electronic soldering flux
	Isocyanates	Epoxy resins
	Platinum salts	Over 100 agents are recognized as causing occupational asthma
Aspirin	Common to all non-steroidal anti-inflammatory agents	Usually non-atopic individuals
		Associated with nasal polyps
(b) Non-specific triggers		
Exercise ⎫ Dry/cold air ⎭	Related to amount of exercise	Common, possibly due to drying of airways
Smoke	Cigarettes	
Air pollutants	Sulfur dioxide ⎫	Related to amount of
Chemicals	Chlorine ⎭	exposure
Emotional stress		
Climatic factors	Temperature changes	
	Fog	
Idiosyncratic factors	Laughter, perfume	

pathogenesis to asthma brought on by a reaction to aspirin (aspirin-sensitive asthma). The debate as to whether asthma is one or several diseases is still unresolved, although recent work demonstrating that the pathology of asthma is essentially the same whatever the clinical presentation has strengthened the argument in favor of the single-disease hypothesis.

One general point about asthma is that it is a disease localized to the airways. It is not associated with other diseases, apart from in some individuals the allergic diseases hay fever and eczema. This suggests that the basic defect in asthma is not due to a generalized abnormality in a particular type of tissue, such as smooth muscle or epithelium, but is a localized problem due to a defect in an airway structure brought about by some airborne environmental stimulus.

One way of classifying asthma is based on the suspected environmental trigger. In this respect it is important to distinguish between those agents that may actually cause asthma, for example by causing an abnormal immune response (specific triggers), and those that aggravate already existing asthma to produce an exacerbation of the disease (non-specific triggers). The response to non-specific triggers is usually related to the amount of exposure. In practice there is a certain amount of overlap between the two. For example, viral infections and exposure to allergens may be responsible for both initiating the inflammatory response that underlies asthma and for aggravating already existing inflammation. *Table 1.1* describes some important triggers for asthma.

1.1.2 Extrinsic vs. intrinsic asthma

Traditionally a fundamental division has been drawn between atopic (extrinsic) and non-atopic (intrinsic) asthmatics. Atopy is the trait whereby some individuals (about 30% of the population) make immunoglobulin E (IgE) against a variety of generally airborne antigens, which because of this relationship to allergic disease are termed allergens. Allergens are generally complex mixtures of large proteins derived from animal and plant dusts. Common allergens include the fecal pellets of the house dust mite (*Dermatophagoides pteronyssinus; D. farinae* in USA), grass pollen, and cat and dog hair (*Table 1.2*). What makes an antigen an allergen has been the subject of intensive study and is discussed in Chapter 6. IgE binds very tightly to high-affinity receptors on the surfaces of mast cells and basophils, and cross-linking of the IgE receptor, through binding of allergen to IgE, results in mast cell degranulation and the rapid release of histamine and other inflammatory mediators. This is the classic type I hypersensitivity response and is most clearly illustrated by the skin prick test, in which allergen is pricked into the skin with a needle and, if the individual is atopic to that allergen (i.e. has made specific IgE against it), a wheal and flare reaction ensues after about 5 min. Indeed, this is the simplest and easiest way to determine if a subject is atopic. Occasionally a

Table 1.2: Common allergens

Type	Example	Comment
Pollens (wind-borne)	Grass Timothy grass (*Phleum pratense*)	Large pollen grains do not easily penetrate to small airways. Responsible for hay fever, summer asthma
	Ragweed (*Ambrosia artemisifolia*)	Equivalent to grass pollen-related disease in the USA
	Tree	Spring hay fever/asthma
	Flowers/weeds	Late summer/autumn
Animal danders	Cat	Common and potent causes of asthma
	Dog	Animal allergens persist for months after departure of pet from the home
	Horse	
	Small animals	Rabbits, hamsters, allergens in urine/feces
House dust mite	*Dermatophagoides pteronyssinus* *Dermatophagoides farinae*	Commonest allergens worldwide. Breed in warm humid conditions. Allergens in fecal pellet
Fungal spores	*Alternara* spp. *Aspergillus* spp. *Cladosporum* spp. *Didymella* spp.	Smaller, more respirable particles than pollen. Decaying vegetation. Late summer/autumn peak
Foods	Egg Milk	Uncommon in adults

skin test is inappropriate, for example if the patient has very bad eczema or is taking anti-histamines which inhibit the skin test reaction. In this case specific IgE can be measured directly using an immunoassay such as a radioallergoadsorbent test (RAST), in which the patient's serum is added to the allergen bound to a solid phase such as a paper disk and the amount of IgE bound quantified by adding radiolabeled IgE. Thus, atopic individuals may be defined as being skin test positive to at least one of a range of common allergens; non-atopic individuals are skin test negative. Asthma is commoner in atopic individuals. The atopic trait also runs in families, and there is evidence that it has an autosomal dominant pattern of inheritance. Atopic asthmatics are termed extrinsic because an allergen coming from outside is thought to be the cause of the asthma.; and non-atopic asthmatics are termed intrinsic because no such outside influence is obviously involved. The two groups of asthma do have different clinical profiles (*Table 1.3*), but there is considerable overlap. In addition, it is

Table 1.3: Intrinsic vs. extrinsic asthma

	Extrinsic	Instrinsic
Age of onset (years)	< 20	> 30
Sex	1.6:1 male:female	1:1 male:female
Total IgE	High	Low
Skin prick test	Positive	Negative
Allergic trigger		
clinically identified	Sometimes	No
Severity	Mild to severe	Generally more chronic and severe

often difficult to identify a clear allergic trigger in many extrinsic asthmatics. Further evidence that the distinction between the two patterns of disease may not be so important is the observation that when IgE levels were corrected for age (blood IgE levels fall off with age) asthma in non-atopic individuals over the age of 55 years was shown to correlate with total IgE concentrations to the same extent as in younger, extrinsic asthmatics. It is therefore questionable whether the division of asthma into two groups has furthered our understanding of the disease. Furthermore, as mentioned above, studies investigating the pathology of asthma have shown very similar changes in the airways whether the asthmatics be extrinsic or intrinsic.

1.1.3 Definition and diagnosis

Although asthma in its characteristic presentation is readily recognized, the variety of clinical patterns of the disease, the lack of a perfect understanding of its pathogenesis and overlap with other conditions have made an exact definition difficult to establish. Asthma is most clearly characterized by episodes of increased airflow obstruction which if sufficiently severe lead to breathlessness and wheeze. The airflow obstruction can vary in severity and pattern from mild, transient episodes of wheeze and chest tightness to severe and prolonged breathlessness at rest. A key feature of asthma is that the severity of airflow obstruction will vary over a relatively short time frame, either spontaneously or as a result of treatment with drugs such as β_2-agonists or anti-inflammatory agents, particularly corticosteroids. An attempt at a consensus definition was made at a Ciba Foundation symposium in 1973, which proposed:

> Asthma refers to the condition of subjects with widespread narrowing of the bronchial airways which changes in severity over short periods of time either spontaneously or under treatment and is not due to cardiovascular disease.

The reference to cardiac disease is because pulmonary edema due to heart failure can lead to variable airflow obstruction (cardiac asthma), which disappears when the heart failure is treated with diuretics. One feature of asthma is an increased sensitivity of the airways to non-specific irritants (bronchial hyperresponsiveness). This feature was given greater prominence in a definition proposed by the American Thoracic Society:

> Asthma is a clinical syndrome characterized by increased responsiveness of the tracheo-bronchial tree to a variety of stimuli. The major symptoms of asthma are paroxysms of dyspnea, wheezing and cough, which may vary from mild and almost undetectable to severe and unremitting (*status asthmaticus*). The primary physiological manifestation of this hyperresponsiveness is variable airflow obstruction. This can take the form of spontaneous fluctuations in the severity of obstruction following broncho-dilators or corticosteroids, or increased obstruction caused by drugs or other stimuli.

This statement, though comprehensive, rather contravenes the dictum that a definition is useful in inverse proportion to its length. The problem with both these definitions is that neither the physiological changes nor the clinical features of asthma are completely specific, being shared by other obstructive airways diseases. Lung diseases can be divided broadly into two categories depending on the site of the disorder: restrictive and obstructive. In this respect the lung can usefully be thought of as an upside down tree without roots. The trunk is the windpipe (trachea); the branches are the airways (bronchi), which divide into ever smaller branches (bronchioles); finally the most distal branches give way to the leaves, which are equivalent to the grape-like bunches of sacs (alveoli), where gas exchange occurs. In general terms obstructive lung diseases affect the bronchi while restrictive lung diseases affect the alveoli and peripheral lung tissue (*Figure 1.2*). The two types of lung disease can be most readily distinguished by simple breathing tests in which the patient is asked to inhale as deeply as possible and then to forcibly expel the air into a machine (spirometer) that measures the amount (forced vital capacity,

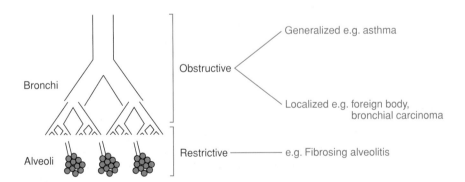

Figure 1.2: Types of lung disease. In very general terms there are two types of lung disease. Obstructive lung diseases such as asthma affect the airways (bronchi), whereas restrictive lung disease affects the alveolar tissue.

FVC) and speed (forced expiratory volume in one second, FEV_1) at which the air is expelled. An additional measure is the top speed that the air achieves on being expelled, the peak expiratory flow rate (PEFR or PEF), which can be measured using a small hand-held meter (peak flow meter). The patterns of changes in lung function seen in restrictive and obstructive lung disease are outlined in *Table 1.4*. The peak flow detects obstruction in the large and medium-sized airways, which are particularly affected in asthma, although there is evidence that the abnormalities occur throughout the bronchial tree. The PF is therefore the most useful and sensitive measure of lung function in asthma and has the advantage of

Table 1.4: Lung function in restrictive and obstructive lung disease

	Obstructive	Restrictive
FEV_1	↓↓	↓
FVC	↓	↓↓
FEV_1–FVC ratio	↓	↑
Peak flow	↓	Normal

↓, decrease; ↑, increase.

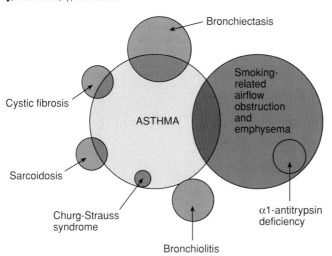

Figure 1.3: Overlap syndromes in obstructive lung disease. There are a number of obstructive lung diseases which in some cases are characterized by an asthmatic pattern of variable airflow obstruction. The relation between the pathogenesis of the variable airflow obstruction in asthma and these other diseases is uncertain. Bronchiolitis is permanent and fixed damage to the small airways, often secondary to a viral infection. α_1-Antitrypsin deficiency is an inherited disease leading to severe emphysema. Emphysema is destruction of the small airways and alveoli generally due to smoking. Churg–Strauss Syndrome is an eosinophilic vasculitic disease associated with asthma. Sarcoidosis is a granulomatous inflammatory disease affecting the lung tissue and sometimes the airways.

being readily measured at home by the patient. Generally a 20% change in airflow obstruction, as measured by either peak flow or FEV_1, is regarded as diagnostic for asthma. Other obstructive lung diseases that have asthmatic features are bronchiectasis (a disease in which the bronchi are damaged by persistent infection), cystic fibrosis (which is a form of bronchiectasis) and chronic obstructive airways disease (COAD; other acronyms include chronic obstructive lung disease, COLD; chronic airflow obstruction, CAO; and chronic obstructive pulmonary disease, COPD), which itself is a spectrum of disease states, usually related to smoking-induced lung damage. The interaction between these various diseases may be illustrated using a Venn diagram (*Figure 1.3*).

1.1.4 Bronchial hyperresponsiveness (BHR)

A cardinal feature of asthma is an increased sensitivity of the airways to non-specific irritants. This is reflected in the way in which irritants such as smoke, dust, cold air and perfume can trigger an asthma attack. The degree of sensitivity of the airways to noxious stimuli can be quantified by measuring the concentration of a non-specific bronchoconstrictor, usually histamine or methacholine, which causes a 20% fall in the FEV_1. This is termed the provocational concentration causing a 20% fall (Pc20). A selection of dose–response curves to histamine is illustrated in *Figure 1.4*.

  The Pc20 of a random population is normally distributed, with asthmatics being clustered at the left-hand end of the normal curve

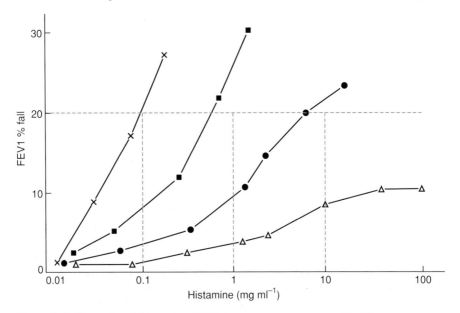

Figure 1.4: Example of histamine Pc20 dose–response curves. X—X, very hyperresponsive subject with brittle asthma; ■—■, moderately hyperresponsive asthmatic; ●—●, borderline between asthmatic and normal; △—△, normal dose–response.

(*Figure 1.5*). A Pc20 of less than 4 mg ml^{-1} methacholine is highly suggestive of asthma. A Pc20 above 8 mg ml^{-1} methacholine is normal, with between 4 and 8 mg ml^{-1} being a gray area. About 5% of a normal population will have a Pc20 of less than 8 mg ml^{-1}. In normal individuals the Pc20 usually plateaus, so that despite increasing the concentration of inhaled histamine no further fall is seen in the FEV$_1$. This plateau is not observed in many asthmatics, particularly those with more severe disease. There is an inverse correlation between the severity of asthma and the Pc20. The Pc20 changes over time broadly in concert with the degree of symptoms. Thus the Pc20 of asthmatics who only get asthma during the hayfever season when exposed to grass pollen will fall during the pollen season and return to more normal values outside the season. The Pc20 can be a useful test in patients in whom the diagnosis of asthma is uncertain and, in addition, is often used in a research context as an objective measure of asthma severity.

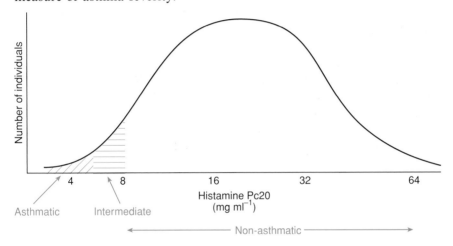

Figure 1.5: Distribution of histamine Pc20 values in the general population.

The cause of bronchial hyperresponsiveness is not clear, though in part it may be due to geometric factors related to wall thickness (discussed in Chapter 2). However, there seems to be a general relationship between airways inflammation and bronchial hyperresponsiveness. Asthmatics in remission who have normal airways pathology are not generally hyper-responsive, whereas asymptomatic asthmatics who do have inflamed air-ways are hyperresponsive. In addition, other lung diseases in which air-ways inflammation is thought to be important, such as chronic bronchitis and bronchiectasis, are associated with airways hyperresponsiveness. Corticosteroids, which are thought to be effective in asthma by suppres-sing airways inflammation, lead to an increase in the Pc20 (i.e. a reduction in bronchial hyperresponsiveness). While it appears that airways inflam-mation is important in revealing a tendency to hyperresponsiveness, there is no clear correlation between the severity of the inflammation and the degree of BHR. For example, in many studies measures of airways inflammation such as numbers of infiltrating leukocytes or mast cells have not correlated very well with the Pc20. Some patients with marked BHR have only mild airways inflammation. It is likely therefore that BHR is dependent on variables other than inflammation alone.

1.1.5 Summary

Asthma is therefore a disease characterized by variable airflow obstruction in which the sufferer is highly sensitive to a variety of airways irritants that readily lead to bronchoconstriction. As is discussed in Chapter 2, the airways obstruction is due to a combination of edema of the bronchial wall, plugging of the lumen with inspissated mucus, and spasm of the bronchial smooth muscle. Underlying these events is airways inflammation (*Figure 1.6*).

1.2 Epidemiology

Asthma is present worldwide. However, there are striking variations in prevalence. In children from the Papua New Guinea Highlands a prevalence of 0.007% has been reported compared with 75% in children under 5 years in the Western Caroline Islands. It is often difficult to determine exact prevalence within populations because of methodological problems. These are mainly concerned with the difficulty in confirming the diagnosis in large population studies. Questionnaires based on symptoms

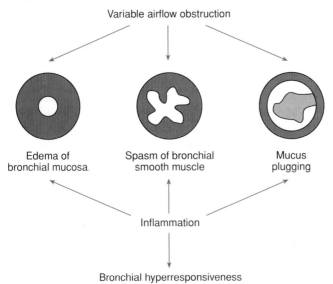

Figure 1.6: Asthma is characterized by variable airflow obstruction caused by a combination of edema, smooth muscle spasm and mucus plugging, which in turn are due to airway inflammation. Airway inflammation is associated with bronchial hyperresponsiveness.

alone such as cough and wheeze are likely to include many non-asthmatics. Ideally, epidemiology studies should include lung function measurements to confirm variability in peak flow or FEV_1, but these are often difficult to undertake. In Britain, asthma in children, based on symptoms and questionnaire, has a current prevalence (number of people with the disease at any one time) of about 10% and a cumulative prevalence (number of people who have ever had the disease) of about 20%. In adults, European studies suggest a current prevalence of about 2–4% based on a diagnosis of asthma made by the investigator or general practitioner and up to 20% based on a history of wheezing episodes. There is evidence from epidemiology studies for both genetic and environmental components to the disease. Geography appears important in that asthma is more prevalent in damp climates, with a low prevalence in dry climates, particularly above 2000 m, possibly because of the inability of the house dust mite to breed at a relative humidity of less than 60%.

In certain areas specific triggering factors which lead to a marked increase in asthma have been defined. For example, in the Sudan an increase in the prevalence of asthma was found to be due to allergy to the green nimitti midge *Cladotanytarsus leuoisi*, and in Barcelona epidemics of acute severe asthma were caused by allergic reactions to soya bean dust released into the atmosphere from ships being unloaded in the docks. In the UK more boys are affected than girls (1.6:1), but this difference is not seen in adults. Immigration studies suggest that a lifestyle associated with developed countries leads to an increased incidence of asthma. For example, children born in India or Pakistan immigrating to Britain have been found to have a lower incidence of asthma than Asian children born in Britain or East African Asian immigrants to the UK who had led a Westernized lifestyle. However, the high prevalence in other under-developed countries suggests that asthma is not the prerogative of a Western lifestyle. Changes in prevalence and severity within a community strongly support the role of environmental factors in the etiology and expression of asthma. One example is the apparent increase in mortality from asthma in the UK in the 1960s, which returned to normal in the 1970s. A similar pattern has occurred more recently in New Zealand. In both cases, and particularly in New Zealand, there is evidence to suggest that potent, long-acting β_2-agonists were responsible.

Another striking example of rapid changes in the prevalence of asthma is shown by the South Fore people of Papua New Guinea. In the 1970s the current prevalence was nil in children and 0.3% in adults. In the 1980s it rose to 0.6% in children and 7.3% in adults. A high incidence of atopy to house dust mite allergen, and high concentrations of house dust mites have been found in blanket dust from these villagers. The blankets have only been introduced relatively recently.

There has also been a suggestion of a general increase in the incidence of asthma and allergic rhinitis in the UK over the last 20 years. It is often difficult to compare studies performed at different times, often using different methods. Part of an observed increase may refer to asthma being diagnosed whereas previously it was referred to as wheeze. However, in the USA, prevalence in one study increased from 5 to 7.6% over a 10 year period in 6- to 11-year-old children. In Finland asthma prevalence amongst conscripts was 0.3% in the 1960s and 1.8% in 1989. Substantial increases in the rates of hospital admission have also been observed in children in the UK, USA and New Zealand.

1.3 Clinical features of asthma

Asthma can vary in severity from occasional attacks of mild wheeziness and breathlessness, to life-threatening episodes that require emergency hospitalization, to chronic debilitating breathlessness that constantly interferes with quality of life. Asthma can vary in severity within an individual so that generally mild asthmatics may have periods when they have more severe symptoms. Sometimes the cause of these changes can be identified: a new pet; pregnancy, which causes a deterioration in 33% of women, improvement in 33% and no change in 33%; or a severe viral cold. More usually no cause is found. Asthma can also remit for months or years and then return for no apparent reason. Disease severity is therefore a continuum measured by degree of symptoms, amounts of treatment required and impairment of lung function (usually peak flow). Clinical features are summarized in *Table 1.5* and detailed below, although division into mild, moderate and severe is to an extent arbitrary.

1.3.1 Mild and moderate asthma

Typically a mild asthmatic will have occasional attacks of wheeziness, often following upper respiratory tract infections or after contact with a known allergen such as cat, dog or horse hair. Often wheeziness appears only during exercise or when in contact with a particularly smoky atmosphere. The individual may occasionally wake at night with cough and chest tightness. The episodes of breathlessness and wheeze will rapidly resolve a few days after the cold has subsided or after contact with the allergen has ceased. These episodes will generally be controlled by intermittent use of inhaled β_2-agonists such as salbutamol or bricanyl, although low doses of inhaled steroids may be required for periods following a cold or during the early summer in seasonal asthmatics. Often disease-free periods may be prolonged and individuals may not regard themselves as having asthma. Examination during attacks may reveal occasional expiratory wheeze on auscultation of the chest and be normal between attacks. Although lung function will be well preserved it would be likely to show variability in peak flow during attacks of asthma and even when the subject is asymptomatic. It is important to note that the ability of an individual to sense loss of lung function varies greatly, with considerable loss not noticed by some people, especially if they lead

Table 1.5: Clinical features of chronic asthma

	Mild	Moderate	Severe
Nocturnal wakening (frequency)	< once per month	< once per week	2–3 times per week
Daytime symptoms	Intermittent mild breathlessness and wheeze	Frequent breathlessness and wheeze, occasionally troublesome	Continuous breathlessness and wheeze
Exercise ability	Unlimited except EIA	Troublesome	Very limited
Effect on lifestyle	Minor	Occasional days off work and limitation in activities	Considerable limitation in all activities
Bronchodilators	Intermittent use, once a day	More than once a day	Frequent use, 4 times a day. Requiring high-dose nebulizer treatment
Inhaled steroids	Occasional periods of use	Regular low/medium-dose inhaled steroids	Regular high-dose inhaled steroids
Oral steroids	No	Occasional courses	Frequent courses, sometimes continuous
Peak flow (% predicted)	> 90%	> 70%	< 60%
Previous admissions	No	Occasional	Frequent

EIA, exercise-induced asthma.

sedentary lives and the loss has occurred over some time. Some asthmatics with only few symptoms may therefore have disproportionate loss of lung function. Mild asthma with intermittent and easily controlled symptoms is more commonly seen in the younger extrinsic type of asthmatic, although there is considerable overlap. Moderate asthmatics have more persistent symptoms, with nocturnal waking, some impairment of activities and marked sensitivity to airborne irritants. They require daily bronchodilators. However, their symptoms are well controlled on modest doses of inhaled steroids and their peak flow is more than 75% predicted normal for age, sex and height. They will rarely, if ever, have severe attacks requiring emergency visits by the GP or admission to hospital. They will not require time off work and with the help of inhaled steroids will be able to lead a normal active life.

1.3.2 Chronic moderate to severe asthma

Patients are continuously aware of their symptoms, and their impaired lung function inhibits their lifestyle because of limited ability to undertake exercise. They may have difficulty holding down a job. It is likely that they will have had asthma without remission for many years and most asthmatics come to terms with their illness although, like all chronic disease, it can lead to depression and anxiety, especially if long-term treatment with corticosteroids has led to side-effects such as bruising, skin thinning and osteoporosis. Some patients will have marked nocturnal symptoms of cough, breathlessness and wheeze, which lead to poor sleep patterns. Although a sign of poor asthma control, nocturnal symptoms are often difficult to eradicate. Examination will often reveal a patient who is mildly breathless on performing fairly modest tasks, such as walking to the clinic or getting undressed. Wheeze may be detected from the end of the examination couch and certainly on auscultation of the chest. However, the patient will not be in distress, and signs of acute severe asthma, which are detailed below, will be absent. Investigations will reveal impaired lung function with a peak flow of less than 75% predicted and often as low as 25% predicted, which should improve following inhalation of β_2-agonists. The patient will be usually be satisfactorily managed with continuous high-dose inhaled corticosteroids and occasional courses of oral corticosteroids during exacerbations, together with inhaled and occasionally oral bronchodilators. In more severe cases continuous oral corticosteroids may be necessary together with high-dose bronchodilators administered through a nebulizer.

1.3.3 Acute severe asthma

Asthma is a life-threatening disease from which between 1000 and 2000 people aged less than 65 die every year in the UK. Death usually occurs in the context of an attack of acute severe asthma. Generally, this occurs against a background of unstable and often undertreated disease, although this is frequently only recognized in retrospect. Instability can be recognized through symptoms such as marked nocturnal wheeze and cough, frequent and increasing requirement for inhaled bronchodilators which have decreasing efficacy, and difficulty taking gentle exercise such as walking upstairs. Severe attacks of asthma can occasionally come on very suddenly, even in someone with previously mild disease. This can occur when allergic individuals suddenly inhale large amounts of the allergen to which they are sensitive. This is seen most dramatically in epidemics of asthma, such as the Barcelona epidemics due to soya bean dust, in which many relatively mild asthmatics suddenly developed severe attacks of asthma.

The acute severe asthmatic will be distressed, breathless at rest and using accessory muscles (neck, shoulder and rib muscles) to force air in and out of the chest. Wheeze may be marked but the chest may be silent, a sinister sign denoting that little air is moving in and out of the lungs and indicating imminent collapse and death. The patient will have difficulty talking in complete sentences due to the effort of breathing and be unable to walk more than a few steps. Examination will reveal a racing pulse, a marked difference between the systolic blood pressure when the patient breathes in and out (pulsus paradoxus), increased respiratory rate and possible cyanosis (the patient's lips and mouth will look deep red or even bluish). Usually, the patient will be hypoxic on measurement of blood gases. The pCO_2 will fall in the early stages of acute severe asthma and will rise with increasing severity. A high normal carbon dioxide level in the presence of hypoxia in acute severe asthma is an ominous indication that respiratory arrest is not far off. Treatment involves the rapid administration of high concentrations of oxygen, large doses of bronchodilators both by inhalation and possibly intravenously, and high doses of corticosteroids. In the most extreme cases the patient may need artificial ventilation until the drugs have time to work. In some cases this may need to be prolonged for several days.

1.4 Childhood asthma

Asthma is the commonest chronic disease of childhood. The undeveloped nature of the infant's lung and particularly the narrowness of the small airways means that small degrees of bronchoconstriction or airways narrowing due to mucosal edema can have a marked effect. Although it has been traditionally thought that children grow out of asthma, this is not true of children with more severe and early-onset disease. Their asthma often persists into adulthood. A large proportion of children with asthma are atopic, and allergy is thought to play an important part in the etiology of childhood asthma. In addition, the relationship between viral infections and exacerbations of asthma is more clear cut than in adults in that an airways viral infection can be more readily documented in association with exacerbations of the disease. Treatment of children with asthma follows the same general principles as with adult asthma, however many infants under 2 years of age respond only poorly to bronchodilators. This may be because mucosal edema is more important at this age than airways narrowing due to spasm of the bronchial smooth muscle.

1.5 Clinical variants of asthma

There are a number of variants of asthma which are interesting from a point of view of pathogenesis. These include types of asthma with specific triggers such as occupational asthma, exercise-induced asthma, aspirin-induced asthma and asthma that is resistant to treatment with corticosteroids.

1.5.1 Glucocorticoid-resistant asthma

Corticosteroids are the mainstay of the treatment of chronic asthma either by the oral route or more usually by inhaler. Corticosteroids are effective in asthma because of their anti-inflammatory activities, an area that is discussed in more detail in Chapter 7. A subset of patients who appear clinically to have asthma, in that they are non-smokers with greater than 20% increase in peak flow after inhaled bronchodilators and no other evidence of chest disease, do not respond to corticosteroids. This can be established by asking asthmatics to keep a daily peak flow chart while treating them for 2 weeks with 0.5 mg kg^{-1} prednisolone, an oral glucocorticoid. Over 90% of asthmatics will improve their peak flow readings by more than 20%, but between 1 and 5% will have no improvement in either their symptoms or their lung function. These asthmatics tend to be at the more severe end of the disease spectrum. It has been shown that some of these patients have a defect in their biochemical response to glucocorticoids. For example, T-lymphocyte proliferation is usually effectively inhibited by glucocorticoids, however proliferation of T lymphocytes from glucocorticoid-resistant asthmatics is unaffected by physiological doses of glucocorticoids.

1.5.2 Aspirin-sensitive asthma (ASA)

Up to 10% of chronic severe asthmatics are intolerant of aspirin. Aspirin ingestion in these subjects causes bronchospasm, rhinoconjunctivitis and in severe cases anaphylaxis and even death. These symptoms can occur within minutes or hours. ASA is often associated with nasal polyposis and a marked peripheral blood eosinophilia. Subjects are usually non-atopic. This is a class effect of cyclo-oxygenase inhibitors so it also occurs with other non-steroidal anti-inflammatory drugs. The diagnosis is based on clinical history supplemented, if necessary, by an aspirin challenge. The cause of ASA is unknown, however because it appears to be a non-immunological effect related to the cyclo-oxygenase inhibitory activity of aspirin it is thought to be due to an abnormality in arachidonic acid metabolism. Arachidonic acid forms the substrate for two major classes of cell-derived inflammatory mediators: the leukotrienes, generated by the activities of an enzyme called lipoxygenase, and the prostaglandins, generated by the lipoxygenase enzyme. There is evidence for abnormal production of arachidonic acid-derived mediators in ASA, although the fundamental defect is still unclear. An interesting aspect of ASA is that patients can be desensitized by administration of regular aspirin, starting at low doses in patients who are highly sensitive.

1.5.3 Occupational asthma

As is the case with general asthma triggers, asthma triggers in the workplace can be divided into those that are non-specific irritants acting to aggravate pre-existing asthma and specific agents that can actually cause asthma. The term occupational asthma is usually restricted to specific triggers. The overall prevalence of occupational asthma is not known, although over 100 agents have been described to cause workplace-related disease. The major causes of occupational asthma are listed in *Table 1.6*. Occupational asthma remains underdiagnosed, and rates in the UK may be as high as 63 per million. Diagnosis is based on a careful job

Table 1.6: Some agents that cause occupational asthma

Agent	Chemical nature	Occupation
Urine of laboratory animals	P	Experiment scientist
Grain mites	P	Farm workers
		Grain storage handlers
Flour	P	Bakers
Green coffee beans	P	Coffee bean handlers
Bacillus subtilis	P	Washing powder manufacture
Plicatic acid (western red cedar)	LMC	Lumberjack (British Columbia)
Colophony (pinewood resin)	LMC	Soldering
Acid anhydrides	LMC	Epoxy resins
Isocyanates	LMC	Manufacture of polyurethane foam, paints, varnishes
Reactive dyes	LMC	Textile industry
Platinum salt	LMC	Platinum manufacture

P, protein; LMC, low molecular weight chemical.

history, detailed peak flow recordings including work and rest periods, and if necessary, challenge with the offending agent.

Many occupational agents appear to be allergens stimulating specific IgE production either to the agent itself or, in the case of low molecular weight chemicals, the agent bound to albumin (in this case the agent is acting as a hapten). Smoking is associated with increased risk of developing specific IgE to a workplace agent. With many agents (e.g. plicatic acid) there is no evidence of specific IgE production and non-atopics are at equal risk as atopics in developing the asthma. While amount of exposure is likely to be important in whether a worker develops occupational asthma, only a relatively small proportion of people exposed to a known agent will develop asthma. An interesting feature of occupational asthma is that it often persists for several years after a person is no longer exposed to the agent involved. Thus, at an average of 4 years after exposure had ceased, 60% of people with red cedar wood asthma caused by plicatic acid were symptomatic. This illustrates that the initiating stimulus in asthma may be distinct from the events that control persistence of the inflammatory response.

1.5.4 Exercise-induced asthma (EIA)

Up to 80% of asthmatics will bronchoconstrict after vigorous exercise or after hyperventilating cold dry air. Bronchoconstriction occurs within 5–10 min, is generally not severe and regresses spontaneously after 30–90 min. Often in mild, usually young, asthmatics EIA is the only symptom. It has been observed that EIA is more likely if patients are breathing in cold rather than warm air, suggesting that cooling of the airways is responsible. However, when the temperature of the air was varied but the water content kept the same asthmatics had similar degrees of EIA. EIA occurred in dry air, suggesting that it was drying of the airways that was responsible possibly by making the bronchial mucosa hypertonic. Hypertonicity can cause mast cell degranulation both *in vivo* and *in vitro*, and mast cell-derived mediators such as histamine have been shown to be released during EIA. Anti-histamines are effective in partly inhibiting EIA, and a drug called disodium cromoglycate (Intal), which prevents mast cell degranulation, is also effective . There is therefore good evidence that EIA is due, at least in part, to mast cell degranulation. After asthmatics have exercised there is a refractory period of 1–2 h, during which about 50% of subjects will have a less than 50% degree of bronchoconstriction during a second period of exercise. This occurs even if the first exercise was performed in warm air and did not provoke asthma. The mechanism of refractoriness is uncertain, although it may be related to the release of protective prostaglandins, as the refractory period is blocked by indomethacin. In any case the refractory period can be used therapeutically, for by undertaking a pre-exercise routine in warm air EIA can be avoided or at least blunted.

1.5.5 Allergic bronchopulmonary aspergillosis (ABPA)

This is a syndrome characterized by asthma, peripheral blood eosinophilia and fleeting shadows on the chest X-ray. The exact incidence of ABPA is not clear but it probably occurs in about 1% of asthmatics. It is caused by a vigorous immune response to *Aspergillus fumigatus* (although it has been described with other fungi) which colonizes the airways without invasion. In addition to ABPA, *Aspergillus* can cause several types of lung disease. These include allergen-induced bronchoconstriction secondary to inhalation of fungal spores, a fungal ball called an aspergilloma that colonizes old lung cavities usually due to healed tuberculosis, a chronic necrotizing pneumonia, and an invasive disseminated infection seen in immunocompromized individuals. ABPA is diagnosed if asthma is present together with chest X-ray shadowing and an immunological profile consisting of a high total and *A. fumigatus*-specific IgE, IgG precipitating antibodies in the serum, a raised eosinophil count, and *A. fumigatus* cultured in the serum. An important feature of ABPA, when it has become established, is the presence of bronchiectasis, often more prominent in the upper lobes, probably caused by persistent obstruction of the large airways by inspissated mucus. In severe cases this can lead to extensive lung damage and respiratory failure. Treatment aimed at avoiding this compli-cation often necessitates long term oral corticosteroids. The reasons why some asthmatics develop ABPA is unknown. As *A. fumigatus*-specific IgE is always present, a skin prick test to an extract of the fungus is a simple screening test: if the skin test is negative ABPA is excluded; if positive, as occurs in about 10% of asthmatics, further investigations can be undertaken.

1.6 Management and treatment of asthma

The principles of asthma management have been alluded to above and are summarized in *Table 1.7*. Initially a firm diagnosis should be made and the severity of the disease established. This is done by a combination of a careful history and assessment of lung function including peak flow monitoring over a period of weeks. Exacerbating and triggering factors should be elicited and where possible avoided. For example, allergen avoidance such as removal of feather pillows and possibly the family pet may be considered appropriate. A careful job history may reveal potential occupational triggers for asthma. Once the pattern and severity of disease have been determined the aim of treatment should be to minimize the effects of the disease on a person's lifestyle, to prevent severe attacks of asthma, and to maintain lung function as close as possible to a person's predicted normal value. Recently a set of guidelines for the management of both chronic and acute severe asthma was drawn up for the UK by the British Thoracic Society (BTS) in conjunction with the National Asthma Campaign and the King's Fund and internationally by a panel of experts under the auspices of the National Institutes for Infectious and Allergic Diseases in Bethesda, USA. The BTS guidelines for the treatment of chronic asthma are summarized in *Table 1.8*. The general principle of both

Table 1.7: Principles of asthma management

(1) Confirm diagnosis (> 20% reversibility in peak flow in absence of other lung disease)
(2) Identify triggers and give advice on avoidance
(3) Assess severity
(4) Assess patient attitude to disease and involve in asthma education
(5) Prescribe appropriate treatment with careful attention to inhaler device and observance of guidelines for treatment of chronic asthma

Table 1.8: BTS guidelines on chronic asthma

Step 1
Occasional β_2-agonists
Step 2
β_2-Agonists and inhaled steroids, 200–800 µg day^{-1} (twice daily dose) or cromoglycate/nedocromil
Step 3
β_2-Agonists + high-dose inhaled steroids, 800–2000 µg day^{-1} via spacer. In the occasional patient unable to tolerate high-dose inhaled steroids consider an inhaled long-acting β-agonist or theophylline
Step 4
β_2-Agonists + high-dose inhaled steroids + trial of one or more of theophylline, an inhaled long-acting β-agonist, inhaled Atrovent, Oxitropium, a β_2-agonist tablet, high-dose inhaled bronchodilators via a nebulizer
Step 5
Above + regular oral prednisolone

Review every 3–6 months. Step down where possible

these sets of guidelines is that treatment should be matched to severity of disease with the emphasis on anti-inflammatory drugs to help prevent symptoms rather than overreliance on bronchodilators, which only provide short-term relief. However, both types of treatment obviously have a complementary role to play in asthma management.

1.7 Asthma and the environment

Although there is evidence for a genetic component to asthma, the wide variations in the prevalence of asthma and the lack of complete concordance between identical twins (i.e. asthma occurs in both twins in only about 30% of cases) suggest that environmental factors play a major part in whether a genetically susceptible individual gets the disease. Some environmental triggers were listed in *Table 1.1*, where they were divided into specific and non-specific agents, the former having the potential to cause asthma as well as aggravate pre-existing disease. The most important specific triggers are viral infections and allergens together with the occupational agents discussed above. In addition, there is increasing evidence that air pollutants, particularly from cars, are important in both causing and aggravating asthma.

1.7.1 Allergens

Allergens are complex foreign proteins, usually from animals, plant pollens or house dust mites (HDMs), which in a large proportion of people stimulate the production of IgE antibodies directed against them. The commonest allergens were listed in *Table 1.2*. The route of entry of allergens is mainly across mucosal surfaces, namely the respiratory and intestinal epithelia. It has been well recognized for many years that allergens can cause asthma in atopic individuals, and this is the basis for the allergen challenge model of asthma described below. However the importance of allergens in causing asthma is still a subject of controversy. In many extrinsic asthmatics a clear relationship between allergen exposure and disease is difficult to obtain and many people who are atopic do not get asthma. If 30–50% of a population are atopic as defined by a positive skin test to at least one of a range of common allergens, about half will manifest some form of allergic disease and about one-quarter will have some symptoms of asthma at some time, although this may be only occasional mild wheeze in the grass pollen season. It is often difficult to recognize that an allergen is causing asthma because exposure is low level and continuous, causing a chronic inflammatory state rather than sudden episodes of airways obstruction. However, when HDM-sensitive asthmatics were moved from houses with high levels of HDM allergen to a hospital bed with low levels of HDM allergen there was a considerable improvement in both symptoms and bronchial hyperrespon-siveness. In addition, the increase in asthma in parts of Papua New

Guinea referred to above can clearly be related to increased exposure to HDM. There is also a good correlation in random population studies between atopy and both bronchial hyperresponsiveness and asthma. Atopy in young children is an important risk factor for the later development of asthma. This does not prove that atopy causes asthma but, taken together with our current understanding of the pathogenesis of asthma, it provides compelling evidence for the importance of allergens in the disease. The combination of skin test positivity to an allergen together with a history of exposure to that allergen is therefore sufficient evidence to advise asthmatics to take avoidance measures even if a symptomatic relationship is not obvious. The problem is that avoidance is very difficult. Patients are often reluctant to part with pets, and pollens, house dust mites and fungal spores are so ubiquitous as to be difficult to avoid. It is difficult to reduce levels of HDM allergen to below the threshold that causes problems, and even obsessive cleaning, barrier methods and the use of acaricides to kill the mite has proved disappointing so far. In trying to eradicate allergens from the home it should be noted that allergens from pets can remain at high levels for months after the pet has departed unless vigorous spring cleaning is undertaken. Nonetheless, advising common-sense measures to reduce allergen exposure is part of the routine management of asthma. The molecular structure of allergens and why they cause such a characteristic immune response is of obvious interest and is discussed in Chapter 6.

1.7.2 Viruses

It is well recognized, especially in children, that an attack of asthma is preceded by an upper respiratory tract infection (a cold) which then 'goes onto the chest'. Colds are caused by viruses rather than bacterial infections. A number of viruses have been implicated in this response by the demonstration of an increase in antibodies against the virus and by culturing the virus from nasal secretions (*Table 1.9*). In one study of 16 children aged 3–11 who experienced 61 episodes of asthma over a year, 42 episodes were associated with symptomatic respiratory infection and in 24 a virus was directly implicated, with rhinovirus being the commonest cause. Not all viral infections cause attacks of asthma. In one study only 4 of 21 asthmatics experimentally infected with rhinovirus developed a significant fall in their lung function. There is a suggestion that viral

Table 1.9: Viruses associated with exacerbations of asthma

Virus	Approximate percentage of infections
Rhinovirus	60
Coronavirus	25
Respiratory syncytial virus	10
Parainfluenza virus	5

infections, particularly with respiratory syncytial virus (RSV), in infancy can lead to asthma later in life. Of 130 children admitted to hospital in the first 5 years of life with RSV lower respiratory tract infection, 42% (compared with 19% of controls) had future episodes of wheezing together with a threefold increase in the incidence of bronchial hyperresponsiveness.

The mechanism of action of viruses in triggering asthma attacks is not clear. In part they may be acting as allergens triggering a specific IgE response. For example, RSV-IgE titers in 79 children with documented RSV infection were highest in those children with evidence of airways obstruction. In addition, a virus will provoke a cell-mediated immune response as well as being potentially cytotoxic to the bronchial epithelium. In this respect the observation that viral infections increase bronchial hyperresponsiveness in non-asthmatic humans, possibly through provoking an airway inflammatory response, is of interest.

1.7.3 Air pollution

The apparent increase in both the prevalence and severity of asthma over the last two decades has paralleled the increase in the number of cars. This has led to the suggestion that air pollution may be responsible for causing or aggravating asthma. There are two main types of air pollution derived from the burning of fossil fuels such as oil and coal: (i) particulates and sulfur dioxide; (ii) photochemical smog. The known effects of air pollutants on asthma are summarized in *Table 1.10*.

Sulfur dioxide (SO_2). It is well established from major air pollution episodes in the middle of the twentieth century in Europe and the USA that sulfur dioxide and particulate air pollution are detrimental to respiratory health and can exacerbate and possibly cause asthma. This is also illustrated by the high incidence of lung disease, including asthma, in

Table 1.10: Relationship between air pollutants and asthma

Air pollutant	Effect on asthma
Sulfur dioxide (SO_2)	Bronchoconstriction
	Asthmatics 5–10 fold more sensitive than non-asthmatics
Particulates	Not tested
Nitrogen dioxide (NO_2)	Bronchoconstriction
	Variable effect
	No clear-cut difference between asthmatics and normal subjects
Acid aerosols	Similar to NO_2
Ozone (O_3)	Airway inflammation
	Reduced lung volumes
	Increased BHR
	No obvious difference between asthmatics and non-asthmatics

polluted parts of Eastern Europe. Considerable efforts have been made with some success to improve air quality with regard to SO_2 and particulates, although concentrations that could potentially aggravate asthma are still regularly found in the UK. Asthmatics are hyperresponsive to SO_2. Thus inhalation of SO_2 by asthmatics under controlled laboratory conditions causes bronchoconstriction at much lower concentrations than in non-asthmatics. Although the wheeziness is transient and readily reversible in the mild asthmatics on whom these studies have been done, in more severe asthmatics it might be expected that inhalation of SO_2 would have more serious effects. SO_2 appears to be working more as a non-specific trigger in that it does not cause increased bronchial hyper-responsiveness and affects non-asthmatics only at high concentrations.

Photochemical smog. The pollutants derived from car exhausts are numerous and include nitrogen oxides, hydrocarbons, heavy metals and ozone. Ozone is a secondary product of car exhausts formed from nitrogen oxide in the presence of hydrocarbons and sunlight. Ozone is a highly reactive molecule that can cause oxidant-mediated damage to a wide variety of plant and animal tissues. This includes the respiratory epithelium, to which it is toxic at the relatively low concentrations found in the ambient air. Increased concentrations of ozone in the lower atmosphere (as opposed to the upper atmosphere, where it is being depleted) have become commonplace in Europe, including the UK, in recent years. Ozone at concentrations found in UK air can cause reduced lung function, airways inflammation and increased bronchial hyperresponsiveness. There is also evidence that it increases the risk of atopic disease by acting as a co-stimulant for the generation of IgE antibodies to common allergens. The evidence for ozone being partly responsible for the increased prevalence of asthma in the UK is far from conclusive, but it appears to have profound effects on both asthmatic and normal lungs at concentrations found in ambient air.

1.8 Models of asthma

In many ways it is difficult to investigate the pathogenesis of asthma by studying clinical disease alone. Recruitment of subjects may be difficult, the disease may be too severe and it is difficult to control for aspects of the disease, such as drug treatment, which may affect the results of any study. In addition, the events that initiate and limit the asthmatic process may be hard to discern in on-going disease. For these reasons various models of asthma both in animals and humans have been established. The problem with any model of asthma is that it is studying only a limited aspect of the disease and may give misleading information. This is particularly true of animal models in view of the fact that few if any animals get asthma as a natural disease. Most models of asthma are in fact models of inflammation caused by exposure to allergens. This makes the assump-

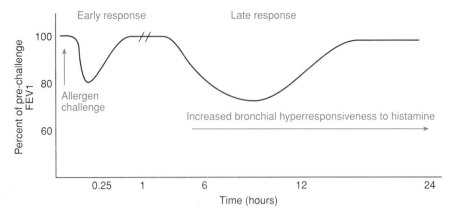

Figure 1.7: The response to inhaled allergens in sensitized individuals. About 40% of subjects get a late response that is associated with increased BHR and is regarded as a model for chronic asthma.

tion that asthma is similar in pathogenesis to allergic inflammation. The basic model is exposure of an atopic individual to a dose of allergen to which they are sensitized sufficient to cause a clinically obvious reaction. This can be done in the skin, nose and lungs. In the skin the clinical response is an initial wheal and flare reaction followed, if the dose of allergen is large enough, by a delayed or 'late response', which is both more florid and prolonged and consists of swelling, discomfort and redness. In the lung a corresponding pattern is observed. There is an initial fall in lung function, which returns to normal after an hour, followed in about half the subjects by a late response, which again is more prolonged and associated with the development of bronchial hyperresponsiveness (*Figure 1.7*). In the nose the initial reaction is characterized by sneezing, mucus production and nasal blockage. A late response is less discernible in the nose. Animal models follow basically the same pattern, only in most cases the animal has to be specially sensitized to make specific IgE. An exception to this are wild-caught monkeys, some of which have been naturally sensitized by infection to parasite antigens. The pathology of the late response has many features in common with asthma, which has led investigators to suggest that the early response more closely represents the acute asthmatic response whereas the late response resembles chronic asthma. A comparison between allergen challenge and clinical asthma is made in *Table 1.11*. Allergen challenge in the lung is a convenient and safe test when performed in experienced hands and has been extensively used in the development of anti-asthma drugs. However, it has a relatively poor record in this respect in that many drugs that are effective in blocking the early and late response do not perform well in real asthma. One reason for this may be because the allergen challenge model emphasizes the role of the mast cell. There is good evidence that the early and, to a lesser extent, late response are the result of mast cell-derived mediators. However, there

Table 1.11: Comparison of allergen challenge with clinical asthma

	Early response	Late response	Clinical asthma
Prolonged obstruction	No	Yes	Yes
Increased BHR	No	Yes	Yes
Airways inflammation	No	Yes	Yes
Inhibited by inhaled steroids	No	Yes	Yes
Inhibited by disodium cromoglycate (Intal)	Yes	Yes	Partially
Inhibited by anti-histamines	Partially	No	No

is increasing evidence, discussed in Chapter 4, that the mast cell may not be such a central cell in the pathogenesis of asthma as was once thought. An alternative model to allergen challenge is exercise-induced asthma. This can be readily performed and is safe and reproducible. However, exercise appears to be a non-specific trigger that causes only short-term bronchoconstriction without airways inflammation and as such is of limited interest from a point of view of pathogenesis.

Further reading

General books on asthma: clinical features and basic mechanisms

Barnes, P.J., Rodger, I.W. and Thompson, N.C. (Eds) (1992) *Asthma: Basic Mechanisms and Clinical Management*, 2nd Edn. Academic Press, New York.

Clark, T.J.H., Godfrey, S. and Lee, T.H. (Eds) (1992) *Asthma*, 3rd Edn. Chapman & Hall, London.

Holgate, S.T. and Church, M.K. (Eds) (1992) *Allergy*. Gower Medical Publishing, London.

Middleton, E., Reed, C.E., Ellis, E., Adkinson, N.F., Yunginger, J.W. and Busse, W.W. (Eds) (1993) *Allergy: Principles and Practice*, 4th Edn. Mosby, St Louis.

Weiss, E.B. and Stein, M. (Eds) (1993) *Bronchial Asthma. Mechanisms and Therapeutics*, 3rd Edn. Little, Brown & Co., Boston.

Historical aspects

Ellul-Micallef, R. (1976) Asthma: a look at the past. *Br. J. Dis. Chest*, **70,** 112–116.

Keeney, E.L. (1964) The history of asthma from Hippocrates to Meltzer. *J. Allergy*, **35,** 215–226.

Definition of asthma

American Thoracic Society Committee on Diagnostic Standards (1962) Definition and classification of chronic bronchitis, asthma and pulmonary emphysema. *Am. Rev. Respir. Dis.*, **85,** 762.

Anon. (1988) Airflow limitation – reversible or irreversible? (Editorial). *Lancet*, **1,** 26–27.

Ciba Foundation Guest Symposium (1959) Terminology, definitions and classification of chronic pulmonary emphysema and related conditions. *Thorax,* **14**, 286.

Ciba Foundation Study Group No 38 (1971) *Identification of Asthma.* Churchill Livingstone, Edinburgh.

Bronchial hyperresponsiveness (BHR)

Cockcroft, D.W. and Hargreave, F.E. (1990) Airway hyperresponsiveness: relevance of random population data to clinical usefulness (Editorial). *Am. Rev. Respir. Dis.,* **142**, 497.

Cockroft, D.W., Berscheid, B.A. and Murdock, K.Y. (1983) Unimodal distribution of bronchial responsiveness to inhaled histamine in a random human population. *Chest,* **83**, 751.

Cockcroft, D.W., Killian, D.N., Mellon, J.A.A. and Hargreave, F.E. (1977) Bronchial reactivity to inhaled histamine: a method and clinical survey. *Clin. Allergy,* **7**, 235.

Holgate, S.T., Beasley, R. and Twentyman, O.P. (1987) The pathogenesis and significance of bronchial hyperresponsiveness in airways disease. *Clin. Sci.,* **73**, 561–572.

Kamm, R.D. and Drazen, J.M. (1992) Airway hyperresponsiveness and airway wall thickening in asthma (Editorial). *Am. Rev. Respir. Dis.,* **145**, 1249.

O'Byrne, P.M., Hargreave, F.E. and Kirby, J.G. (1987) Airway inflammation and hyperresponsiveness. *Am. Rev. Respir. Dis.,* **136**, S35.

Page, C.P. and Gardiner, P.J. (Eds) *Airway Hyperresponsiveness: is it Really Important for Asthma?* Blackwell Scientific Publications, Oxford.

Woolcock, A.J., Salome, C.M. and Yan, K. (1984) The shape of the dose–response curve to histamine in asthmatic and normal subjects. *Am. Rev. Respir. Dis.,* **130**, 71.

Epidemiology

Anderson, H.R. (1989) Is the prevalence of asthma changing? *Arch. Dis. Childh.,* **64**, 172–175.

Asher, M.I., Patlemore, P.K. and Harrison, A.C. (1988) International comparisons of the prevalence of asthma symptoms and bronchial responsiveness. *Am. Rev. Respir. Dis.,* **138**, 524–529.

Bousquet, J. and Burney, P. (1993) Evidence for an increase in atopic disease and possible causes. *Clin. Exp. Allergy,* **23**, 484–492.

Burney, P.G.J., Chinn, S. and Rona, R.J. (1990) Has the prevalence of asthma changed? Evidence from the national study of health and growth 1973–1986. *Br. Med. J.,* **300**, 1306–1310.

Clifford, R.D., Radford, M., Howell, J.B. and Holgate, S.T. (1989) Prevalence of respiratory symptoms among 7 and 11 year old schoolchildren and association with asthma. *Arch. Dis. Childh.,* **64**, 347–355.

Fitzgerald, J.M., Sears, M.R., Roberts, R.S., Morris, M.M., Fester, D.A. and Hargreave, F.E. (1988) Symptoms of asthma and airway hyperresponsiveness to methacholine in a population of Canadian schoolchildren. *Am. Rev. Respir. Dis.,* **137,** 285.

Gergen, P.J., Mullally, D.I. and Evans, R. (1988) National survey of prevalence of asthma among children in the United States 1976–1980. *Pediatrics,* **81,** 1–7.

Clinical features of asthma

Chan-Yueng, M. (1990) Occupational asthma. *Chest,* **98** (Suppl.), 148S.

Corrigan, C.J., Brown, P.H., Barner, N.C., Tsai, J.-J., Frew, A.J. and Kay, A.B. (1991) Glucocorticoid resistance in chronic asthma: activation of peripheral blood T-lymphocytes in glucocorticoid resistant asthmatics and a comparison of the in vitro inhibitory effects of glucocorticoids and cyclosporin A. *Am. Rev. Respir. Dis.,* **144,** 1026–1032.

Douglas, N.J. (1993) Nocturnal asthma. *Thorax,* **48,** 100–102.

Giraldo, B., Bumethal, M.N. and Spink, W.W. (1969) Aspirin intolerance and asthma: clinical and immunological study. *Ann. Intern. Med.,* **71,** 479–496.

Mapp, C.E. *et al.* (1988) Persistent asthma due to isocyanates. A follow up study of subjects with occupational asthma due to toluene diisocyanate (TDI). *Am. Rev. Respir. Dis.,* **137,** 651–655.

Meredith, S.K., Taylor, V.M. and McDonald, J.C. (1991) Occupational respiratory disease in the United Kingdom 1989. *Br. J. Industr. Med.,* **48,** 292.

Wardlaw, A.J. and Geddes, D.M. (1992) Allergic bronchopulmonary aspergillosis: a review. *J. Roy. Soc. Med.,* **85,** 747–751.

Management of asthma

BTS/NAC/King's Fund (1993) Guidelines on the management of asthma. *Thorax,* **48** (Suppl.), S1–S24.

Asthma and the environment

Cameron, K. and Maynard, R. (1992) A new look at the health effects of air pollution. *Health Trends,* **24,** 82–85.

Colloff, M.J., Ayres, J., Carswell, F. *et al.* (1992) The control of allergens of dust mites and domestic pets: a position paper from the BSACT. *Clin. Exp. Allergy,* **22,** 52.

Lippman, M. (1989) Health effects of ozone. A critical review. *J. Am. Pollut. Control Assoc.,* **39,** 672–695.

Pattermore, P.K., Johnston, S.L. and Bardin, P.G. (1992) Viruses as precipitants of asthma symptoms. 1. Epidemiology. *Clin. Exp. Allergy,* **22,** 325–336.

Wardlaw, A.J. (1993) Air pollution and asthma. *Clin. Exp. Allergy,* **23,** 81–106.

Warner, J.A. (1992) Environmental allergen exposure in homes and schools. *Clin. Exp. Allergy,* **22,** 1044–1045.

Chapter 2

The pathology of asthma

2.1 Introduction

Until recently the pathological changes characteristic of asthma had not
been well defined. Most studies were based on the pathology of asthma
deaths and were for obvious reasons anecdotal and involved small
numbers of patients in whom clinical features were often poorly
documented. Studies were generally uncontrolled and were undertaken
on patients who were at the very severe end of the disease spectrum and
therefore atypical of the majority of asthmatics. Over the last 10 years it
has been appreciated that, with appropriate precautions, fiber-optic
bronchoscopy can be safely undertaken to obtain samples from the
airways of mild to moderate asthmatics. As a result, a number of carefully
controlled studies have been performed, leading to an increased
understanding of the pathological changes in asthmatic airways. Despite
their limitations, autopsy studies provide a basic understanding of the
pathology of asthma, which has been complemented rather than
contradicted by later studies using the fiber-optic bronchoscope. Before
describing the pathological features of asthma, a brief outline of the
structure of the normal human lung and airways will be given.

2.2 Structure of the airways

2.2.1 Lung embryology

The lung originates from the foregut, appearing as an epithelial bud at the
caudal end of the laryngeal groove on the 26th day after ovulation. The
bud, derived from the endoderm, forms the epithelium of the airways and
alveoli. It becomes invested in mesenchyme from the mesoderm. This
mesenchymal tissue develops into the connective tissue, cartilage, smooth
muscle and vessels of the lung. Very early in development nerve fibers
arising in the ectoderm migrate into the mesenchyme. By the 16th week
the bronchial tree has developed as far as the terminal bronchioles. By 26

weeks the lungs have developed sufficiently to support life although the full complement of adult alveoli does not develop until about the age of 8 (*Figure 2.1*).

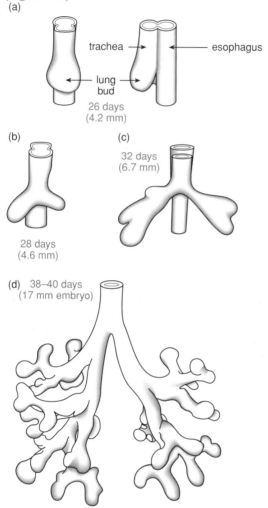

(a)

trachea ——— esophagus

lung
bud

26 days
(4.2 mm)

(b)

(c)

32 days
(6.7 mm)

28 days
(4.6 mm)

(d)   38–40 days
     (17 mm embryo)

Figure 2.1: Schematic representation of the development of the human lung. (a) The trachea can first be identified as a bud arising from the anterior end of the foregut which will become the esophagus (shown from the front and side). (b and c) By 4 weeks the right and left main bronchi start to appear. (d) In the 7-week-old fetus the lobar bronchi can be identified. Reproduced from Pare and Fraser (1983) with permission from W.B. Saunders.

2.2.2 Structure of the adult lung

The windpipe, or trachea, subdivides initially into the two main bronchi, which then subdivide into ever smaller branches until they reach the terminal bronchi, from which the alveoli arise (*Figure 2.2*). The alveoli form grape-like bunches at the end of the bronchi. This unit of alveoli and

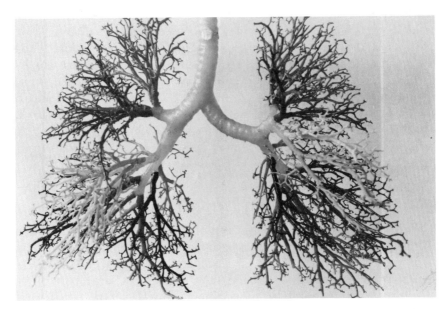

Figure 2.2: A model of the lung, demonstrating the branching structure of the airways. Photographed by Peter Fleissig with permission from Professor B. Corrin (National Heart and Lung Institute, Brompton Hospital, London).

airway is called a respiratory acinus, and it is here that gas exchange occurs. In the thin walls of the alveoli the air comes into intimate contact with the capillaries of the pulmonary circulation, where the blood is reoxygenated on its way to the left side of the heart and the systemic circulation. The human adult has between 200 and 600 million alveoli with the combined surface area of a tennis court (196 m²), making the lungs a highly efficient organ for gas exchange.

The lower airway starts below the larynx and different parts of the airways are defined according to their structure and order of division (*Table 2.1*). The trachea bifurcates at the level of the fifth thoracic vertebra into the right and left main bronchi. The left main bronchus runs for 5 cm before subdividing into left upper and lower lobe bronchi. On the right the upper lobe bronchus comes off almost immediately and then the bronchus

Table 2.1: Airway terminology

Bronchi	All airways which have cartilage in their walls (except the trachea)
Bronchioles	Airways that come after the bronchi
Terminal bronchioles (TBs)	Bronchioles just proximal to the first order of RBs
Respiratory bronchioles (RBs)	Bronchioles from which alveoli arise
Respiratory acinus	Comprises the TB with succeeding (usually three generations) RBs and orders 2–9 of alveolus ducts and sacs. It is 1 cm in diameter and forms the respiratory unit of the lung

intermedius subdivides into middle and lower lobe bronchi. Lobar divisions are followed by segmental and subsegmental divisions. This tree-like branching continues until, after between 8 and 13 divisions from the trachea, the bronchi lose their cartilage and become bronchioles. From the smallest bronchi, which are about 1 mm in diameter, there are 3–4 further subdivisions before the terminal bronchioles are reached, which then divide into the respiratory bronchioles. The cross-sectional area of the airways at the level of the trachea is about 2 cm^2. This increases to about 14 cm^2 at the level of the smallest bronchi and 80 cm^2 at the terminal bronchioles. Thus, maximum resistance to airflow occurs in the larger airways.

2.2.3 Microscopic structure of the airways

The airways consist of a surface epithelium resting on a very thin basement membrane composed of proteins called laminin, collagen and fibronectin (*Figure 2.3*). These are members of a family of extracellular matrix proteins, so called because they make up a large part of the structure of the extracellular tissue. Blood vessels, nerves, mucus cells, resident cells and epithelium are all supported by these fibrillar proteins, which form a mesh-like stroma in which cells reside. Immediately beneath the basement membrane is a 100-µm-deep region rich in blood vessels, fibroblasts and leukocytes supported by the extracellular matrix proteins fibronectin, vitronectin and collagen. This region is called the lamina propria. Together with the epithelium, this forms the mucosa. Beneath the mucosa is the submucosa, consisting primarily of mucus-secreting glands together with cartilage plates and bronchial smooth muscle.

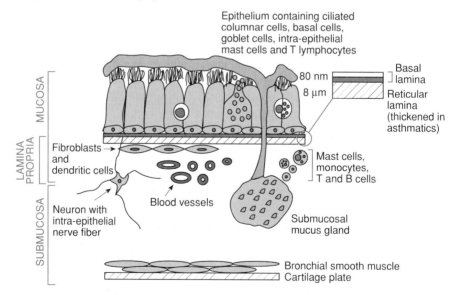

Figure 2.3: Schematic representation of the microscopic structure of the normal human airway illustrating the major cellular components.

Table 2.2: Airway defense mechanisms

(1)	Cough reflexes
(2)	Ciliary activity of the bronchial epithelium
(3)	Secretion of mucus, immunoglobulins, protective enzymes and mediators
(4)	Cellular immune responses
(5)	Protective epithelial barrier

2.2.4 The epithelium

The lining of the entire respiratory tract is continuous with the skin and with the lining of the gut from which it is derived embryologically. The airways, as well as transporting air to and from the alveoli, have other roles, including warming and moistening of the air, protection against infection through a vigilant immune system and removal of inhaled foreign material (*Table 2.2*). The bronchial epithelium has traditionally been regarded as pseudostratified (i.e. all cells rest on the basement membrane but not all reach the airway lumen). However, most of the ciliated columnar cells that make up the majority of the epithelium rest on a layer of basal cells, which are firmly attached to the basement membrane. The ciliated cells have 200–300 cilia, each beating about 1000 times per minute in a cranial direction. Secretions from the mucus glands form a carpet of viscous mucus, which picks up any inhaled debris and is swept along by the cilia to the main airways, where it is expectorated (*Figure 2.4*). The importance of the cilia is illustrated by diseases such as Young's Syndrome, an inherited disease in which cilial function is abnormal, which leads to recurrent lung infections and eventually bronchiectasis. There are a number of different cell types found in the bronchial epithelium, including several different types of epithelial cell, of which the ciliated cell is the most prominent (*Table 2.3*). In addition, nerve fibers that control cough and bronchoconstrictor reflexes pierce the basement membrane and lie between epithelial cells.

2.2.5 Epithelial cell junctions

The epithelium is held together by three types of junction (*Table 2.4*). These junctions have a complex structure (*Figure 2.5*). The tight junctions normally make the epithelium impermeable to the passage of fluids, ions and macromolecules, although following irritation the junction becomes permeable to molecules of molecular mass less than 40 kDa. Transport of molecules across the epithelium appears to involve an active cell process requiring energy. Adhesion between basal cells and columnar cells is mainly through desmosomes, which are complex symmetrical structures derived from constituents of two adjacent cells to form a sort of 'spot weld' between cells. Adhesion between basal cells and the basement membrane is mediated through hemidesmosomes, which contain one of the integrin receptors, $\alpha_4\beta_6$. Integrins are a large family of heterodimeric

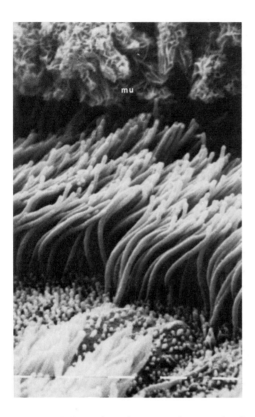

Figure 2.4: Scanning electron micrograph of normal airway epithelium showing the cilia. Each cilium is about 5 μm high and is thought to beat in a low-viscosity perciliary fluid layer at about 1000 times per minute, moving the overlying mucus (mu) only by its tip. × 7000. Courtesy of Dr Peter Jeffery, National Heart and Lung Institute, Brompton Hospital, London.

Table 2.3: Cell types in the bronchial epithelium

(a) Epithelial cells	
Cilated cell	Cilia are 6 μm long and have minute terminal hooklets that aid movement of overlying mucus sheet
Mucus cell	Contains mucin, a sialin-rich glycoprotein. Number increased by smoking
Serous cell	Rare in adult human airway (function unknown)
Clara cell	Non-ciliated. Occur in terminal bronchioles
Dense-core granulated (DCG) cell	Rare; granules contain amines and peptides such as bombesin, which may influence vascular and bronchial tone and mucus secretion
Basal cell	Electron-dense cytoplasm rich in cytokeratin
(b) Migratory cells	
Intraepithelial lymphocyte	May occur singly or in aggregation of lymphoepithelium similar to Peyer patches (aggregated lymphoid tissue in the gut), in which case it is called BALT (bronchial-associated lymphoid tissue). BALT is scanty in humans.
Intraepithelial mast cells	Up to 2% of epithelial cells

Table 2.4: Types of epithelial junction

Type	Location	Function
(1) Tight (zonula occludens) and intermediate (zonula adherens)	Apicolateral surface of epithelial cells	Adherence between cells Barrier to bulk flow of fluid, ions and macromolecules
(2) Desmosomes and hemidesmosomes (spot junctions; maculae adherens)	Between cells and between basal lamina and epithelial cells	Adherence
(3) Nexus or gap junctions	Between cells	Cell-to-cell communication

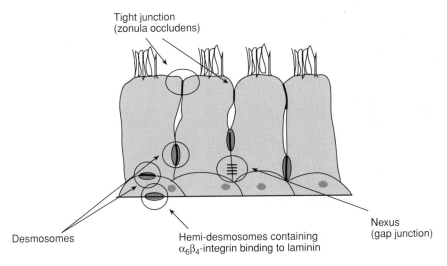

Figure 2.5: Location of different types of epthelial junction in the airway epithelium. After Montefort *et al.* (1992).

(i.e. two different protein chains make up the receptor) glycoprotein membrane receptors. They are the principal cellular receptors for extra-cellular matrix proteins and are also important in a number of cell-to-cell functions. They are described in more detail in Chapter 3. Other integrin receptors have been localized to the epithelium although their function is as yet unclear. So far no major differences in epithelial integrin expression between normal and asthmatic subjects have been demonstrated.

2.2.6 Basement membrane and lamina propria

The epithelium adheres to a basement membrane, which consists of a basal lamina (the true basement membrane) composed of type IV collagen, laminin and fibronectin and a deeper reticular lamina made up of fibrillar collagen of types III and V and fibronectin.

These two components can only be distinguished using electron microscopy. The basal lamina is approximately 80 nm thick and the underlying reticular layer 8 μm thick. It is this second component that is thickened in asthma and other inflammatory conditions of the lung. The components of the basement membrane are derived from fibroblasts, which lie just beneath it. Airway fibroblasts have a distinct character and are termed myofibroblasts because they contain contractile elements in their cytoplasm. Also lying in this region are dendritic cells. These cells constitutively express class II HLA receptors (see Chapter 3) and are highly efficient at presenting antigen to T cells, a key event in the immune response to antigen. In normal individuals the lamina propria is populated by resident mast cells, lymphocytes and monocytes together with small numbers of neutrophils. Eosinophils are rarely seen.

There are a large number of blood vessels in this region. The airways have a very rich vascular network supplied by the bronchial arteries, which in turn derive from the descending aorta and the intercostal and mammary arteries. They therefore have a blood supply distinct from the alveoli, which are supplied by the pulmonary circulation.

2.2.7 Submucosa

The submucosa comprises mainly mucus glands, beneath which lie smooth muscle and cartilage. The glands are described as tubuloalveolar, and from the body of the cell containing the mucous or serous acini and tubules a collecting duct runs towards the epithelium, where it becomes narrow and ciliated before opening out onto the epithelial surface. The mucus secretions that line the airway are therefore derived from both epithelial and submucosal glands. The bronchial muscle completely encircles the intrapulmonary bronchi internal to their supportive cartilage plates.

2.2.8 Airway smooth muscle

There are three main types of muscle in animals: *skeletal*, which has a striated appearance and is under the control of the voluntary nervous system; *cardiac*, which is striated but under the control of internal pacemakers as well as the non-voluntary (autonomic) nervous system; and *smooth muscle*, which has a non-striated appearance and is regulated by the autonomic nervous system. Bronchial muscle is smooth muscle. Smooth muscle cells can be individually supplied with nerves, each behaving as a separate unit (*multi-unit* type, e.g. the iris). This type of muscle does not contract spontaneously. Alternatively, there can be well-developed communications between cells at gap junctions, which allow a signal to be rapidly transmitted throughout the muscle tissue. This *single-unit* type is seen in the muscle of the gut, uterus and ureters and is associated with continuous slow contractions. The bronchial muscle appears to be of the multi-unit type, at least in normal individuals.

The cholinergic arm of the autonomic nervous system, which uses acetylcholine as a neurotransmitter, causes contraction of the bronchial smooth muscle. In addition to its response to neurogenic stimuli, bronchial muscle can be stimulated to undergo relaxation or constriction in response to inflammatory mediators, some of which have been implicated in asthma, such as leukotriene C_4 and prostaglandin D_2, which are discussed in detail in Chapter 5.

Smooth muscle contraction is invariably associated with an increase in the concentration of free intracellular calcium. Stimulation of the cell membrane leads to an initial release of calcium from intracellular stores in the sarcoplasmic reticulum, which is associated with the initiation of contraction and is followed by an influx of calcium from the extracellular medium. This influx of calcium leads to phosphorylation of cytoplasmic myosin, which then binds to actin. These two proteins, which have a fibrillar structure, then slide along each other, which results in shortening of the cell. The intracellular events leading to contraction are complex and have many features in common with the processes that lead to leukocyte activation, which are discussed in Chapter 3.

One of the fundamental abnormalities in asthma leading to airway obstruction and hyperresponsiveness is the increased bulk and contraction of the airway smooth muscle. Little is known about the cause of this increase in the amount of smooth muscle in asthma or the way in which the smooth muscle functions in the disease, in large part because of its inaccessibility.

2.2.9 Innervation of the airways

The lung is richly supplied with nerves, which through the motor or delivery arm (efferent nerves) control bronchial smooth muscle tone, blood supply and mucus gland secretion, being either excitatory or inhibitory. There are three types of efferent innervation to the lung.

(1) A sympathetic nerve supply (adrenergic). As well as the sympathetic nervous system, adrenergic mechanisms also include β_2-adrenergic receptors on bronchial smooth muscle (β_1-receptors are present on cardiac muscle) and circulating catecholamines such as epinephrine, which stimulate these receptors. Adrenergic stimulation results in bronchodilation, and drugs that stimulate β_2-receptors (β_2-agonists) such as salbutamol (Ventolin) and terbutaline (Bricanyl) are the mainstay of relief of bronchoconstriction in asthma.
(2) A parasympathetic nerve supply (cholinergic), stimulation of which causes bronchoconstriction. Drugs that block cholinergic receptors (anti-cholinergics) such as ipratropium bromide (Atrovent) are also effective bronchodilators in asthma.
(3) A non-adrenergic, non-cholinergic (NANC) supply that contains a number of peptide neurotransmitters with a range of functions of potential relevance to asthma, which are discussed in Chapter 5.

Bronchial smooth muscle is directly innervated only by the broncho-constrictor cholinergic pathway. However, β-blockers used in the treatment of hypertension and heart disease, which block both β_1- and β_2-adrenergic receptors, cause bronchoconstriction in asthmatics but not in normal individuals. This suggests that background β-receptor stimulation is important in asthmatics.

The sensory or receptive (afferent) nerve supply comprises type I receptors involved in cough and detection of noxious stimuli, type II receptors involved in pulmonary stretch reflexes and type III receptors of unknown function present deep in the lung.

2.2.10 Mucus

Normal airway mucus consists mainly of water (95%) in addition to salts, proteins, glycoproteins including mucin, lipids and proteoglycans. The viscous properties of mucus are thought to be conferred by mucins, which are a family of variable molecular weight proteins with a flexible core densely covered with sugars *O*-linked to serine and threonine. Proteoglycans may also contribute to the viscosity and elasticity of mucus. Submucosal mucus glands are innervated by both cholinergic and adrenergic nerves, with the former being predominant. Vagal stimulation and muscarinic agonists are effective at increasing mucus secretion, as are several neuropeptides and inflammatory mediators. Of importance in asthma is not only the amount of mucus but its viscosity. What controls the composition of mucus is unclear.

2.3 Pathological abnormalities in the airways in asthma

2.3.1 Autopsy studies

Macroscopic pathology. The macroscopic appearance of the lung of the acute severe asthmatic at post-mortem is characterized by hyperinflation as a result of air trapping, due to occlusion of the bronchi by thick plugs of yellow or white sticky, tenacious material which is glossy and opaque (*Figure 2.6*). Because of these plugs, asthmatic lungs, unlike normal lungs, fail to collapse when the chest wall is opened. The airways plugs consist of a protein-rich inflammatory exudate, with mucus, Charcot–Leyden crystals and desquamated aggregates of epithelial cells, lymphocytes and eosinophils. A similar, though less severe, picture is seen in chronic asthmatics who have died of other causes. A few cases of acute severe asthma reveal less evidence of an inflammatory process. In these cases death may have been due to rapid and overwhelming bronchoconstriction, for example due to the inhalation of a large dose of allergen.

Microscopic pathology. The pathological changes seen in asthma death are summarized in *Table 2.5*. These abnormalities are seen throughout the

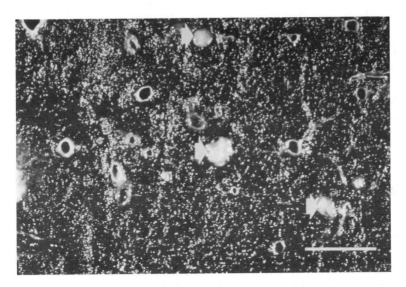

Figure 2.6: Macroscopic appearance of the airways in fatal asthma. A glutinous mucus fills the airways (arrows) and the lung is generally hyperinflated. Courtesy of Dr David Lamb, Department of Pathology, University of Edinburgh, and Allen & Hanburys.

bronchial tree. The most striking and consistent findings are damage to the bronchial epithelium and infiltration of the bronchial wall and lumen by eosinophils and mononuclear cells (*Figure 2.7*). In addition to intact eosinophils large amounts of an eosinophil-derived mediator, eosinophil major basic protein (MBP), have been shown by immunostaining to be deposited in the airways of patients who died from asthma. MBP *in vitro* has been shown to damage bronchial epithelium at concentrations which may be found in asthmatic airways. In asthma it appears that the basal layer of epithelial cells remains attached to the basement membrane, with

Table 2.5: Pathological changes in asthma

Consistent abnormalities
(1) Mucus plugging of the bronchial lumen
(2) Desquamation of the bronchial epithelium
(3) Infiltration of the bronchial mucosa with eosinophils and mononuclear cells
(4) Thickening of the collagen layer beneath the epithelium
(5) Smooth muscle hypertrophy (cell size) and hyperplasia (cell number)
(6) Mucosal edema
(7) Thickening of the bronchial wall

Less consistent abnormalities
(1) Increase in degranulating mast cells
(2) Hypertrophy of mucus glands
(3) Dilatation of the bronchial circulation

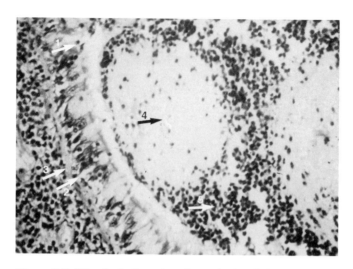

Figure 2.7: Histological section through the airway of a patient who died of asthma showing many of the pathological features characteristic of the disease. Arrowed from 1–5 are: (1) damaged airway epithelium with (2) edema and (3) a thickened collagen layer beneath the basement membrane; (4) a mucus plug blocking the airway; and (5) large numbers of inflammatory cells, particularly eosinophils and mononuclear cells. × 25.

the columnar cells being sloughed off, suggesting that there is a plane of cleavage between the basal and columnar cells. One hypothesis regarding the nature of the underlying susceptibility that leads to asthma is that there is a weakness in adhesion between the basal epithelial cells and the ciliated columnar cells, making the asthmatic epithelium vulnerable to damage by cytotoxic mediators such as MBP. It is loss of surface epithelium that is thought to be responsible for the hyperresponsiveness of asthmatic airways, either through loss of a protective effect and exposure of the epithelial nerve fibers, or through reduced generation of a relaxant mediator normally produced by epithelial cells, although such a factor has not been definitely identified. A recent study by Azzawi *et al.* (1992) has compared the immunohistology of 15 patients who died from asthma with six patients dying of cystic fibrosis and 10 patients dying suddenly from a number of non-inflammatory conditions. The findings of their study are detailed in *Table 2.6*. They confirmed previous studies in finding an increase in the number of eosinophils and T lymphocytes in asthmatic airways. Eosinophils were specific to asthma and not just a feature of chronic lung inflammation as exemplified by cystic fibrosis. Thirteen out of the 15 asthmatics had activated eosinophils in their airways (they used the monoclonal antibody EG2, which stains a secreted form of the eosinophil granule protein, eosinophil cationic protein – ECP – to identify activated eosinophils) compared with none of the 10 sudden death controls. An average of 63 total eosinophils (activated and unactivated) per mm of basement membrane were found in the asthmatics compared

Table 2.6: Immunopathology of asthma deaths (Azzawi *et al.*, 1992)

	Asthma ($n=15$)	Cystic fibrosis ($n=6$)	Sudden death controls ($n=10$)
Total eosinophils	Present in large numbers	Scanty	Very scanty
Activated eosinophils	Present in large numbers, 50% of total	Scanty	Absent
T lymphocytes	Twofold increase over control	Twofold increase	—
B lymphocytes	Equal number as control	Twofold increase	—

with 2.0 per mm in the cystic fibrosis patients and 1.0 per mm in the controls.

As a result of the inflammatory process and smooth muscle hypertrophy there is considerable thickening of the airway wall in patients dying with asthma. This thickening may partly explain bronchial hyperresponsiveness. Wiggs *et al.* (1992) have developed a computer model to investigate the effects of wall thickness on response to broncho-constricting agents. Using direct measurements of airways wall thickness in patients who died from asthma, they have found that their model predicts that smooth muscle constriction in the absence of wall thickening will cause only mild airways obstruction. However, after airway wall thickening, minor increases in smooth muscle constriction could lead to marked increases in airway obstruction. In addition they found that the response of normal subjects to bronchoconstricting agents plateaus, whereas in asthmatics such a response does not occur: they continue to exhibit increasing obstruction with increasing concentrations of bronch-oconstricting agent. This is precisely what has been found in studies comparing the dose–response curves of asthmatic and normal subjects to inhaled histamine and methacholine during measurements of bronchial hyperresponsiveness.

Another consistent feature of the pathology of patients who have died from asthma is marked thickening of the reticular layer of the basement membrane. This is mainly due to increased deposition of collagen type IV. It is non-specific, being also seen with other inflammatory conditions of the airways such as bronchiectasis and chronic bronchitis. The basement membrane is subject to constant remodeling, and whether the thickening is due to increased deposition of matrix protein or inhibition of degradation is not known. In any case it is presumed to reflect a chronic inflammatory stimulus to the fibroblasts that secrete the matrix protein components. This may be equivalent to the fibrotic healing process that occurs in chronic inflammation in other diseases, such as rheumatoid arthritis. Many of the changes in asthma, particularly increased mucus secretion and epithelial desquamation, reflect chronic inflammation at any mucosal surface. The very specific feature of asthma is the presence of eosinophils, which are normally scanty in the airways.

Mucus production in asthma. In health about 10 ml of mucus a day is transported to the larynx and swallowed. No sputum is expectorated. Mucus production in asthma is increased, although to a variable extent. Most asthmatics complain of a dry cough, with only small amounts of sputum being produced. Often the sputum in asthma is green in color because of the presence of degraded leukocytes. This suggests the presence of bacterial infection, although this is unusual in uncomplicated asthma and antibiotics are generally unhelpful. The sputum from asthmatics is often very tenacious, forming viscid plugs that can be difficult to expectorate. Asthmatic sputum has a number of characteristic components (*Table 2.7*). As well as sputum production, evidence that asthma is characterized by increased mucus production is provided by the enlargement of submucosal glands and goblet cell hyperplasia seen at post-mortem. This increased production is presumed to be due to a combination of mucus gland stimulation by neural stimuli and inflammatory mediators. The mucus in asthma appears very viscid. It is not clear whether this is due to increased amounts of plasma proteins including albumin and immunoglobulins, increased amount of mucin or less water relative to solid constituents.

Table 2.7: Constituents of asthmatic sputum

Name	Nature
Curshmann's spirals	Corkscrew-shaped twists of condensed mucus
Creola bodies	Clumps of shed bronchial epithelial cells
Charcot–Leyden crystals	Eosinophil-derived lysophospholipase
Leukocytes	Eosinophils and mononuclear cells
Mucus	Mucin, proteoglycan, lipid, lysozyme, plasma proteins

2.3.2 Fiber-optic bronchoscopy (FOB) studies

Fiber-optic bronchoscopy is a technique in which a flexible scope about the thickness of a pencil and equipped with a light source and viewing lens is passed through the nose or mouth and into the lungs via the larynx. It can then be manipulated to directly visualize the main airways to about the fourth or fifth bronchial division (*Figures 2.8* and *2.9*). This procedure is done under local anesthetic and takes about half an hour. It is a safe and generally well tolerated investigation. It is used to investigate a range of lung disorders, particularly lung cancer. There is a channel in the scope to allow sampling of the airways. Biopsy forceps can be passed down the channel and snips taken of the bronchial lining (endobronchial biopsies).

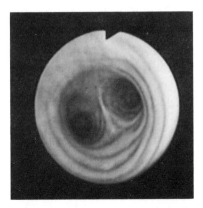

Figure 2.8: View of a normal airway through a fiber-optic bronchoscope showing the cartilaginous rings of the trachea and the sharply demarcated carina which divides right and left main bronchi. In asthma the airway mucosa appears erythematous and edematous.

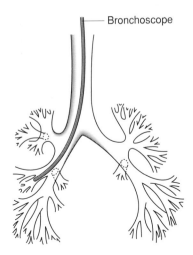

— Bronchoscope

Figure 2.9: Schematic outline of the main airways with an illustration of the fiber-optic bronchoscope being used to sample tissue and fluid from the lungs. Courtesy of Professor A.B. Kay, National Heart and Lung Institute, Brompton Hospital, London.

Alternatively, saline can be instilled into one area of the lung and then aspirated into a bottle. The aspirated fluid contains cells and secretions from the lining of the lung. Small-volume washes (50 ml) sample the airways (bronchial wash), whereas large-volume washes (up to 250 ml) sample the airways and alveoli (bronchoalveolar lavage, BAL). Initially it was thought that FOB would be a hazardous procedure in asthma because of the risk of bronchoconstriction. However, over the last decade a large number of groups have undertaken studies using FOB in mild to moderate asthmatics and it appears to be safe and well tolerated in experienced hands as long as suitable precautions are taken, such as giving nebulized bronchodilators just prior to the procedure. The use of the bronchoscope has allowed detailed, systematic and controlled examination of the pathological changes in asthma of various types and severity. Initially routine histological and electron microscopy techniques were used, but these have now been supplemented by more advanced techniques, such as immunohistology to study cell phenotype in more detail and *in situ* hybridization to look at mRNA expression. Studies have been performed in both steady-state clinical asthmatics as well as in allergic subjects after allergen challenge. Both biopsy studies and BAL studies have been performed. Biopsies are small and often damaged by the forceps but can still yield considerable information. BAL studies allow functional as well as pathological investigations to be undertaken. A summary of the findings of these studies is given below.

Allergen challenge studies. One of the first studies was carried out by de Monchy *et al.* (1985), who demonstrated a correlation between the influx of eosinophils into the airways and the late-phase response to allergen. They found that in subjects who had only an early response there were very few eosinophils in the BAL fluid, but in subjects who developed a late response large numbers of eosinophils were seen. This suggested that eosinophils may be responsible for the development of the late response to allergen challenge. This basic observation has been confirmed and extended by several groups, although in some studies increased numbers of eosinophils were also seen in single early responders. The increase in eosinophil counts after allergen challenge has also been detected in both endobronchial biopsies and BAL fluid after local allergen challenge, where allergen is instilled directly into a segment of the lung through the bronchoscope. In these studies a dramatic increase in BAL eosinophil counts is often observed. Increased numbers of eosinophils are detected at 6 h, are maximal at 24 h and start to decline by 48 h. Increased numbers of airway eosinophils are also observed after challenge with agents that cause occupational asthma, such as plicatic acid and toluene isocyanate. Cromoglycate and glucocorticoids given before allergen challenge inhibit both the late response and the airways eosinophilia.

Some of these studies have shown an increase in the number of neutrophils in the airways, although this has been less consistent and is not affected by cromoglycate or corticosteroids. Mast cells after allergen challenge have a more degranulated appearance. Monoclonal antibodies against various leukocyte membrane receptors have been used to investigate the nature of the inflammatory response in more detail. These studies have shown that, as with asthma deaths, most of the eosinophils are in an activated state ready to secrete their inflammatory mediators. In addition, they have shown increased numbers of activated T lymphocytes in both BAL fluid and biopsies, as defined by expression of the T-cell membrane receptor CD25. The changes seen in association with allergen challenge in the lung are very similar to those seen after allergen challenge in the skin and nose. Although there is a general correlation between the influx of eosinophils and activated T lymphocytes into the airways and the development of the late response, there is some dissociation in the timing in that the inflammatory influx is maximal at about 24 h when the late response has resolved. It is also clear that subjects who do not develop a late response do get an eosinophilia although of lesser degree. It is possible that eosinophilia and the late response are parts of the same phenomenon rather than being directly related, with the fall in lung function being due in large part to airway edema.

As well as the cellular components of the late response, the mediators released after allergen challenge have also been studied by measuring concentrations in BAL fluid, blood and urine. Measurement of mediators in each of these fluids is problematic. The airway secretions in BAL fluid are greatly diluted by the saline inserted, which means that mediators are at very low concentrations. In addition, it is difficult to allow for the variable dilution effect between different samples. Mediator concentrations in serum are very low with contaminating proteins giving high backgrounds. Urine may only contain metabolites of the mediator in question. Some of the mediators released after allergen challenge are summarized in *Table 2.8*. These are generally mast cell derived, consistent with the idea that the allergen challenge response is primarily mast cell driven.

Most recently, *in situ* hybridization, a technique that detects expression of a specific mRNA has been used to determine which cytokine mediators are generated after allergen challenge in both the skin and lung. In this technique a labeled probe is added to frozen tissue sections and allowed to hybridize to complementary sequences of mRNA. Labeling can be performed with a radioactive marker or a dye. A washing step removes unbound probe, with the positive signals that remain indicating positions where the mRNA is being expressed. *In situ* hybridization is a sensitive way of identifying mRNA expression in

Table 2.8: Inflammatory mediators detected after allergen challenge

PGD$_2$	Marked increase in BAL fluid 5 min after local segmental allergen challenge of the airways
LTC$_4$/D$_4$/E$_4$	Variable increase in leukotriene C$_4$ in BAL fluid and plasma in association with early response. Consistent increase in leukotriene E$_4$ in urine
Histamine	Increased amount detected in blood and BAL fluid during early response
Bradykinin	Increased amount in BAL fluid after segmental and aerosolized allergen challenge during early response and 19 h after challenge

tissue. However, it only shows that the gene for a protein has been transcribed and does not show that the protein itself is being produced. There is often a considerable discrepancy between the two events and a complete study needs to show both mRNA and protein being generated. However, it is often difficult to demonstrate the presence of soluble protein mediators in tissue as they are rapidly dispersed and degraded. *In situ* studies have demonstrated that allergen challenge results in increased expression of mRNA for interleukin 5 (IL-5), IL-4, granulocyte–macrophage colony-stimulating factor (GM-CSF) and IL-3, with no increase in expression of gamma-interferon (IFN-γ) and IL-2. These observations have been complemented by similar findings in steady-state asthma, which have also demonstrated that these cytokines are being expressed by T lymphocytes. This pattern of cytokine expression is consistent with activation of a particular subset of T cells called Th2 cells. These findings are discussed in more detail in Chapter 4, but they have given considerable impetus to the idea that asthma is caused by a specific type of lymphocyte response in the airways as a result of allergen exposure.

Steady-state (clinical asthma) studies. The main cellular findings of BAL and endobronchial biopsy studies in clinical asthma are summarized in *Table 2.9*. As can be seen from the table, the pathology of asthma in mild and moderate disease is similar to that seen in asthma deaths, although the changes are generally less severe and less information is obtained about

Table 2.9: Pathological abnormalities in mild and moderate asthma

Eosinophils	Invariably increased in number in both BAL and endobronchial biopsy compared with normal controls. Eosinophils are activated as determined by EG2 staining and expression of the 'activation receptor' CD69. Concentration of basic proteins increased in BAL fluid. Number of eosinophils decreased by treatment with corticosteroids
Lymphocytes	Increased numbers of CD25-positive activated Th2-type T lymphocytes in BAL and endobronchial biopsy. Correlation between numbers of lymphocytes and eosinophils in some studies
Mast cells	Increased number of mast cells in BAL fluid, but this is also seen in other lung diseases. Inconsistent evidence that mast cells in BAL fluid are activated. Morphological evidence of ' degranulation.
Epithelial cells	Number of epithelial cells increased in BAL fluid in asthma. Evidence for epithelial fragility and damage in electron microscopy studies of endobronchial biopsy. Correlation between bronchial hyperresponsiveness and epithelial damage
Other findings	Increased thickness of collagen layer beneath the basement membrane. Increased numbers of monocytes in endobronchial biopsy

the mucus glands and smooth muscle because of the size of the biopsies. As in post-mortem specimens and after allergen challenge, the most consistent and specific finding has been increased numbers of activated eosinophils in both BAL fluid and biopsies. Increased numbers of eosinophils and eosinophil-derived granule proteins are seen even in very mild asthmatics who require only occasional bronchodilators although asthmatics in remission who are asymptomatic and have normal airways responsiveness usually have normal numbers of eosinophils in their airways. There is therefore a close association between bronchial hyperresponsiveness (BHR) and airways inflammation, in that inflammation appears to be required for BHR to develop. However, within an asthmatic population there is generally poor correlation between indices of inflammation, such as eosinophil counts, and severity of BHR as measured by histamine or methacholine Pc20. This suggests that factors other than the severity of inflammation are involved in controlling the degree of BHR. The identity of these factors is yet to be determined. In some studies there has been a better correlation between the degree of epithelial damage in asthma and BHR, but the technical problems of sampling and damage to the epithelium when taking the biopsy make this data difficult to interpret. The link between eosinophils and asthma has been appreciated for many years. Increased numbers of eosinophils have been found in the blood and sputum of asthmatics, and fluctuations in eosinophil counts have been associated with treatment and disease severity. However, an eosinophilia is an inconsistent finding in the blood of asthmatics, and it was not until it was realized that a bronchial eosinophilia is an almost invariable finding in asthma that this cell was placed center stage. At one time eosinophils were thought to be involved in the repair process or as bystander cells, but the realization that they can generate a number of potent mediators that can mimic *in vitro* many of the pathological changes in asthma has led to the hypothesis that eosinophil-derived mediators are primarily responsible for the pathological changes in asthma. The biology of the eosinophil is discussed in Chapter 4.

The mechanisms by which eosinophils are recruited into the lung in asthma is of crucial importance. For many years this was thought to be a mast cell-dependent process, but the observation that activated T cells are found in the airways in asthmatics has switched attention to this cell type. As well as being found in the airways, activated T lymphocytes are found in the blood in acute severe asthma and the numbers decrease with treatment. The role of the T lymphocyte in asthma is also discussed in more detail in Chapter 4.

Above all, FOB studies in asthma have emphasized the inflammatory nature of the disease even in its mildest forms. Although not all clinical types of asthma have been studied by FOB, occupational asthma, intrinsic asthma and extrinsic asthma all show very similar pathological changes. The understanding that the symptoms of asthma are due to underlying inflammation has led to greater emphasis being placed on the treatment of asthma by inhaled glucocorticoid, which are able to dampen the inflammatory response, in the hope that this will prevent attacks of asthma, with relatively less reliance being placed on inhaled bronchodilators. This approach has been reinforced by case studies of patients who have died of asthma, which have suggested that a large proportion of these patients were not on appropriate doses of inhaled corticosteroids. The emphasis on immune suppression and immunomodulation in asthma has led to a number of new potential treatment strategies for asthma which are discussed in Chapter 7.

Expression of adhesion receptors. As discussed in more detail in Chapter 3, leukocyte migration into tissues is controlled by a complex interaction between adhesion receptors on leukocytes and counter receptors expressed by endothelial and epithelial cells. A number of adhesion receptors are highly expressed in normal airways with, in particular, ICAM-1 and E-selectin being constitutively expressed on vascular endothelium. There is some evidence for a modest increase in ICAM-1 and E-selectin expression in intrinsic asthma but not in extrinsic asthma. Expression of ICAM-1 is increased on the bronchial epithelium of asthmatics compared with non-asthmatics, an important observation as ICAM-1 is a receptor for the major group of rhinoviruses. It is possible that upper respiratory tract infections (URTI) cause exacerbations of asthma because the lower airway is vulnerable to infection with viruses as a result of expression of receptors for that virus. VCAM-1 is weakly and variably expressed in both normal and asthmatic airways. There is evidence for increased expression on endothelium of all three of these adhesion receptors after allergen challenge, in both the skin and lung. This suggests that modulation of adhesion receptor expression may be important in controlling the migration of leukocytes into tissue after allergen challenge.

Further reading

Structure of the normal lung

Barnes, P.J. (1990) Neural control of airway function: new perspectives. *Mol. Aspects Med.,* **11,** 351–423.

Barnes, P.J., Baraniuk, J. and Belvisi, M.G. (1991) Neuropeptides in the respiratory tract. *Am. Rev. Respir. Dis.,* **144,** 1289–1314.

Holt, P.G., Schon-Hegrad, M.A. and McMenamin, P.G. (1990) Dendritic cells in the respiratory tract. *Int. Rev. Immunol.,* **6,** 139–149.

Jeffery, P.K., Brewis, R.A.L, White, F.E. and Simpson, V. (1990) Structure of the lung, Section 1. in *Respiratory Medicine* (R.A.L. Brewis, G.J. Gibson and D.M. Geddes, Eds). Balliere Tindall, London.

Pare, J.A.P. and Fraser, R.G. (1983) *Synopsis of Diseases of the Chest.* W.B. Saunders Company, Philadelphia.

Richardson, P.S. and Fung, D.C.K. (1992) Mucus and mucus-secreting cells in asthma, in *Asthma*. (P.J. Barnes, I.W. Rodger and N.C. Thomson, Eds). Academic Press, New York, pp. 157–190.

Stephens N.L. and Seow, C. (1993) Airway smooth muscle: physiology, bronchomotor tone, pharmacology and relation to asthma, in *Bronchial Asthma* (E.B. Weiss and M. Stein, Eds). Little Brown & Co., Boston, pp. 314–332.

Uddman, R. and Sundler, F. (1987) Neuropeptides in the airways: a review. *Am. Rev. Respir. Dis.,* **136**, S3–S8.

Pathology of asthma deaths

Azzawi, M., Johnston, P.W., Majundar, S., Kay, A.B. and Jeffery, P.K. (1992) T lymphocytes and activated eosinophils in airway mucosa in fatal asthma and cystic fibrosis. *Am. Rev. Respir. Dis.,* **145**, 1477-1482.

Dunhill, M.S. (1960) The pathology of asthma with special reference to changes in the bronchial mucosa. *J. Clin. Pathol.,* **13**, 27–33.

Filley, W.V., Itolley, K.E., Kephart, G.M. and Gleich, G.J. (1982) Identification by immunofluoresence of eosinophil major basic protein in lung tissue of patients with bronchial asthma. *Lancet* **2**, 11.

Gleich, G.J., Motojuma, S., Frigar, E., Kephart, G.M., Fujisawa, T. and Kravis, L.P. (1987) The eosinophilic leukocyte and the pathology of fatal bronchial asthma: evidence for pathologic heterogeneity. *J. Allergy Clin. Immunol.,* **80**, 412.

Naylor, B. (1962) The shedding of the mucosa of the bronchial tree in asthma. *Thorax,* **17**, 69–72.

Sabonya, R.E. (1985) Concise clinical study. Quantitative structural alterations in longstanding allergic asthma. *Am. Rev. Respir. Dis.,* **130**, 289–292.

Immunopathology of asthma

Azzawi, M., Assoufi, B., Collins, J.V., Durham, S., Kay, A.B., Bradley, B., Jeffery, P.K., Frew, A.J., Wardlaw, A.J. and Knowles, G. (1990) Identification of activated T-lymphocytes and eosinophils in bronchial biopsies in stable atopic asthma. *Am. Rev. Respir. Dis.,* **142**, 1407–1413.

Beasley, R., Roche, W.R., Roberts, J.A. and Holgate, S.T. (1989) Cellular events in the bronchi in mild asthma and after bronchial provocation. *Am. Rev. Respir. Dis.,* **139**, 806–817.

Bentley, A.M., Menz, G., Storz, C.H.R., Robinson, D.S., Bradley, B., Jeffery, P.K., Durham, S.R. and Kay, A.B. (1992) Identification of T lymphocytes, macrophages and activated eosinophils in the bronchial mucosa in intrinsic asthma. *Am. Rev. Respir. Dis.,* **146**, 500–506.

Bousquet, J., Chanez, P., Lacoste, J.Y. *et al.* (1990) Eosinophilic inflammation in asthma. *New Engl. J. Med.,* **323**, 1033–1039.

Jeffery, P.K., Wardlaw, A.J., Nelson, F.C., Collins, J.V. and Kay, A.B. (1989) Bronchial biopsies in asthma: an ultrastructural quantification study and correlation with bronchial hyperreactivity. *Am. Rev. Respir. Dis.,* **140**, 1745.

Laitinen, L.A., Heino, M., Laitinen, A., Kava, T. and Haahtela, T. (1985) Damage of the airway epithelium and bronchial reactivity in patients with asthma. *Am. Rev. Respir. Dis.,* **131**, 599–606.

Metzger, W.J., Zavala, D., Richerson, H.B., Moseley, P., Iwamota, P., Monick, M., Sjoersdsma, K. and Hunninghake, G.W. (1987) Local allergen challenge and bronchoalveolar lavage of allergic asthmatic lungs. Description of the model and local airway inflammation. *Am. Rev. Respir. Dis.,* **135**, 433–440.

de Monchy, J.G.R., Kauffman, H.F. and Verge, P. (1988) Bronchoalveolar eosinophilia during allergen-induced late asthmatic reactions. *Am. Rev. Respir. Dis.,* **139**, 1383.

Montefort, S., Herbert, C.A., Robinson, C. and Holgate, S.T. (1992) The bronchial epithelium as a target for inflammatory attack in asthma. *Clin. Exp. Allergy,* **22**, 511–520.

Ohashi, Y., Motojima, S., Fukuda, T. and Makino, S. (1992) Airway hyperresponsiveness, increased intracellular spaces of bronchial epithelium and increased infiltration of eosinophils and lymphocytes in bronchial mucosa in asthma. *Am. Rev. Respir. Dis.,* **145**, 1469–1476.

Robinson, D.S., Hamid, Q., Ying, S., Tsicopoulos, A., Barkans, J., Bentley, A.M., Corrigan, C., Durham, S.R. and Kay, A.B. (1992) Predominant Th2 type bronchoalveolar lavage T-lymphocyte population in atopic asthma. *New Engl. J. Med.,* **326**, 298–304.

Roche, W.R., Beasley, R., Williams, J.H. and Holgate, S.T. (1989) Subepithelial fibrosis in the bronchi of asthmatics. *Lancet,* **1**, 520–524.

Wardlaw, A.J., Dunnette, S., Gleich, G.J., Collins, J.V. and Kay, A.B. (1988) Eosinophils and mast cells in bronchoalveolar lavage fluid in mild asthma: relationship to bronchial hyperreactivity. *Am. Rev. Respir. Dis.,* **137**, 62–69.

Wiggs, B.R., Bosken, C., Pare, P.D. and Hogg, J.C. (1992) A model of airway narrowing in asthma and in chronic obstructive pulmonary disease. *Am. Rev. Respir. Dis.,* **145**, 1251–1258.

Chapter 3

Inflammation in asthma I. Principles of the inflammatory response

3.1 Introduction

Asthma is characterized by airways inflammation. Inflammation is the response of the host to tissue damage, which may have a variety of causes including infection, physical injury or toxic chemicals. The aim of the inflammatory response is to limit the tissue damage, remove the cause and then repair the damaged organ (*Figure 3.1*). The characteristics of any particular inflammatory response will depend on the type, severity and persistence of the initial insult, the organ involved and the effectiveness of repair. The inflammatory response is usually divided into: (1) an acute reaction in which the cycle of initial insult, inflammatory response repair and resolution occurs over a period of a few days or weeks and, (2) a chronic inflammatory reaction in which there is continuation of the response over weeks, months or years. In practice, the microscopic events in the acute and chronic phases of an inflammatory response are broadly similar, although acute inflammation is often characterized by a predominance of neutrophils in the tissue compared to mononuclear cells (macrophage/monocytes and lymphocytes), and chronic inflammatory responses are usually considered to cause more tissue destruction.

The inflammatory response is characterized by dilation of the blood vessels at the site of injury (vasodilation), increased permeability of the blood vessels so that protein leaks out into the tissues, causing edema, and emigration of leukocytes from the blood vessels into the extravascular space. These events are caused by chemical mediators generated as part of the inflammatory process. They lead to the cardinal features of an inflammatory response, tumor, rubor, calor and dolor, described by Celsus (30 BC–AD 30), to which Virchow (1821–1902) added loss of

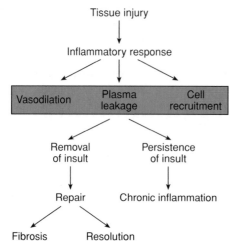

Figure 3.1: Outline of the events following tissue injury. An inflammatory response is induced which leads to removal or neutralization of the causative agent allowing repair of any tissue damage. Whether repair is complete, leading to full resolution, or results in a fibrotic reaction, with permanent tissue damage, will depend on the nature and severity of the initial insult and the organ involved. If the causative agent persists or the inflammatory process becomes self-perpetuating, chronic inflammation ensues which often leads to more pronounced tissue damage and a greater likelihood that repair will lead to fibrosis and scar formation.

function. *Table 3.1* suggests how these features can be related to the inflammatory response in asthma. Many features of the inflammatory response, such as control of vascular tone and permeability, are common to all types of inflammation, and readers are referred to a textbook of pathology for a general description of these events. Some aspects of inflammation, such as activation of the complement cascade, are not, on current evidence, relevant to asthma and will not be discussed in this

Table 3.1: Inflammation

Macroscopic feature	Microscopic feature	Relationship to asthma
Swelling (tumor)	Edema due to vascular leakage and leukocyte accumulation	Edema and cellular infiltration of the bronchial wall
Redness (rubor)	Vasodilation	Vasodilation of bronchial capillaries
Heat (calor)		and venules
Pain (dolor)	Stimulation of pain fibers	Bronchial hyperresponsiveness
Loss of function	Tissue damage	Bronchoconstriction

chapter. The distinctive features of the inflammatory response in asthma are its apparent basis in a disordered immune response to inhaled antigen and the emphasis of leukocyte-mediated events in its pathogenesis. This chapter therefore focuses on describing the way in which the immune system responds to antigen in a specific manner and the processes involved in leukocyte migration and function.

3.2 Cells of the immune system

Circulating white blood cells (leukocytes) form the major cellular component of the immune response supported by cells resident in the tissues. These include endothelial cells, as well as other structures such as mucus glands, smooth muscle and the local neural system (*Table 3.2*). The exact role of a cell can best be determined when there is an isolated defect in the function of that cell. This happens relatively rarely and so the precise function of some cell types, for example natural killer (NK) cells, in the immune response is not clear. In addition there is a degree of overlap so that if one cell type is functioning abnormally its role can be adopted by other cells.

Leukocytes were originally described according to their staining properties, which in turn were based on the mediators stored within their cytoplasmic granules (*Figure 3.2*). Thus, eosinophils were so named because they stained avidly with the acidic dye eosin (eosinophil granule contents are very basic). They were then classified according to their

Table 3.2: Cellular components of the immune system

	Major proposed function in immune response
(a) Circulatory cells	
T lymphocytes ⎫ B lymphocytes ⎭	Antigen-specific responses, host defense against viral infections
NK cells	Unknown
Monocytes	Antigen presentation, phagocytosis and degradation of foreign antigens
Neutrophils	Host defense against bacteria
Eosinophils	Host defense against helminthic parasitic infections
Basophils	Unknown
Platelet	Fragments of bone marrow-derived cells (megakaryocytes) mainly involved in coagulation but possibly having a role in inflammatory cascade
(b) Resident cells	
Dendritic cells	Antigen presentation
Fibroblast	Secretion of matrix proteins
Endothelial cells	Gateway to the extravascular tissues
Mast cells	Major cell involved in type I hypersensivity reactions
Epithelial cells	Protective barrier
Macrophage	Derived from blood monocyte, phagocytosis of foreign antigen

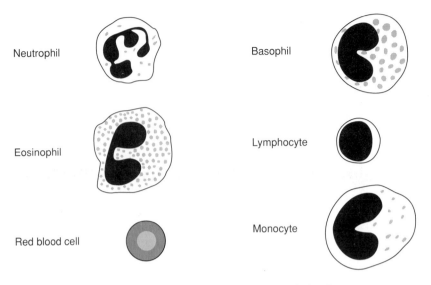

Neutrophil

Basophil

Eosinophil

Lymphocyte

Monocyte

Red blood cell

Figure 3.2: Schematic representation of leukocyte and platelet structure.

structural properties into granulocytes (i.e. granule-containing cells: neutrophils, eosinophils, basophils and macrophages) and mononuclear cells (monocytes and lymphocytes) or, alternatively, according to their functional properties into phagocytes (i.e. cells that readily engulf small particles) and non-phagocytes. Neutrophils and monocytes are phagocytic. Lastly, leukocytes are often grouped according to their developmental lineage, with cells being regarded as myeloid and non-myeloid. Myeloid cells are neutrophils, macrophages and eosinophils.

3.3 Membrane receptors

Membrane-bound receptors are the senses of the cell, through which it communicates with the extracellular environment. They are therefore central to the function of the cell. Most membrane-bound receptors are glycoproteins (i.e. they consist of a protein core with sugar groups attached at various sites) and have a characteristic structure with long extracellular domains, a short hydrophobic domain that anchors the protein in the membrane, and variable-length cytoplasmic domains through which the receptor transmits signals into the cell (*Figure 3.3*). Variations on this theme include receptors which are anchored in the membrane by a lipid (phosphatidylinositol glycan, PI linkage), in which case they lack a cytoplasmic domain, and receptors which span the membrane a number of times. Receptors may be single chain or comprise two or more chains. If both chains are the same the receptor is said to be homodimeric; if different, heterodimeric. Often one chain is unique and one chain is shared by other closely related receptors, as is the case with the integrin superfamily of adhesion receptors discussed below. Receptors may cluster together to form a functional unit, of which the T cell–

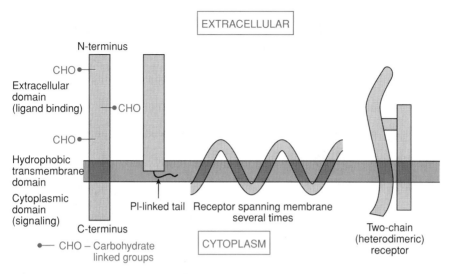

Figure 3.3: Outline of the structure of different receptor motifs.

receptor complex also discussed below is a good example. Like all proteins, receptors are folded into a three-dimensional structure. It is this structure that is recognized by other proteins (counter-structures or ligands), which bind to the receptor because of complementarity of shape and the electric charge of the adjacent amino acids. Counter-structures can be soluble mediators such as histamine, antibodies or reciprocal receptors on other cells. Engagement of a ligand to its receptor usually results in a signal being sent into the cell via a complex signaling pathway, which can result in the cell becoming either stimulated or suppressed. Receptors are called a variety of names, usually associated with their function or the manner in which they were discovered. In many cases they will also have a CD number (cluster of differentiation). CD numbers have been agreed by an international workshop. Most receptors have been found by raising monoclonal antibodies against various cell types. Where two or more antibodies recognize the same molecule on the cell surface the molecule is given a CD number. CD numbers usually, though not always, define a single protein structure. Any one receptor molecule can have a number of different names, which can be confusing. For example, an extremely important receptor on neutrophils, eosinophils and macrophages is the heterodimeric, two-chain integrin CD 11b/CD18. This is also termed α_M/β_2 because of its integrin family membership, Mac-1 because it was first described as a macrophage receptor, Mo-1 for the same reason (monocyte receptor) and complement receptor 3 (CR3) because it is the receptor for the complement fragment C3bi. Membrane receptors, like other proteins, can be grouped together according to structural criteria based on their primary nucleotide sequence. A number of gene families have been described, including the integrin superfamily, the immunoglobulin superfamily and the rhodopsin family of G protein-linked receptors, which are involved in recognition of chemotactic agents. Grouping within a gene family suggests the molecule has originated from a primordial gene which has mutuated over the eons. Often different genes have come together so that different domains within a receptor may be related to different gene families. This is of more than evolutionary interest for common structural features often suggest common functions and ligands.

One of the largest and most diverse gene family of receptors is the immunoglobulin superfamily. The receptors involved in antigen recognition (the T-cell antigen receptor, the B-cell immunoglobulin receptor and the major histocompatibility complex – MHC – receptors) are all members of this family as well as immunoglobulin itself.

3.4 Antigen recognition

The basis for recognition of foreign proteins (antigens) by the immune response is receptors expressed by T and B lymphocytes that can recognize antigens in a unique fashion. T cells are the cornerstone of cellular immunity, an immune reaction based on direct cellular interactions, whereas B cells produce antibodies (the humoral response). B cells require help from a subset of T cells, termed T helper cells, to produce antibody. There are a number of different subsets of T cells classified mainly according to expression of various membrane receptors. The major T-cell subsets are illustrated in *Figure 3.4*.

The acquired immune system must have the capacity to recognize, in a specific fashion, myriad different types of foreign protein structure. It is

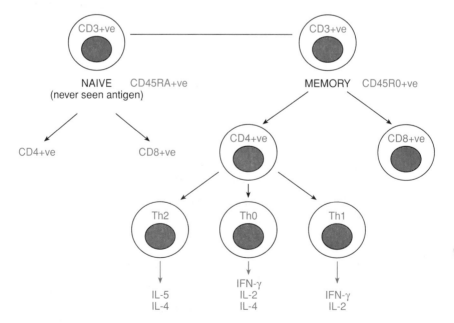

Figure 3.4: Major T-lymphocyte subsets.

able to do this through antigen recognition structures on B cells and T cells that are subtly different on each individual cell so that each cell recognizes a different and unique antigenic structure. The T-cell structure is called the T-cell antigen receptor and the B-cell structure is a modified form of immunoglobulin anchored in the membrane.

3.4.1 The T-cell antigen receptor

The T-cell antigen receptor is composed of an antigen recognition structure and receptors involved in signal transduction. Together they constitute a receptor complex called CD3 (*Figure 3.5*). The antigen recognition structure is heterodimeric, being comprised of two distinct protein chains, an α- and β-chain, each with a molecular mass of about 40–50 kDa (an infrequent subset of T cells has similar though distinct γ- and δ-chains). These chains are disulfide linked (i.e. covalently linked by sulfide bonds), transmembrane glycoproteins. Each of the chains has two immunoglobulin-like domains. The distal N-terminal domain is highly variable and is responsible for the unique antigen recognition properties of the receptor. This variability is due to rearrangement of the different genes which make up the variable region during development of the lymphocyte repertoire in the fetus. The proximal domain has a constant structure. At the cell surface the α/β heterodimer is non-covalently associated with five other peptide chains which together make up the CD3 complex. The chains are called CD3-γ, -δ, -ε, -ζ-ζ, and -ζ-ῆ. These chains are responsible for trans-ducing the signal resulting from antigen binding to the α/β chains into the cell, resulting in cytokine release and cell

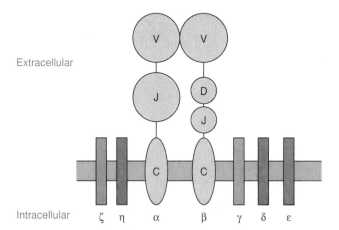

Figure 3.5: Schematic outline of the structure of the CD3 T-lymphocyte–receptor complex showing the α- and β-chains of the antigen recognition element and the other chains involved in signal transduction. The variable (V), joining (J) and diversity (D) regions of the α- and β-chains make up the antigen binding regions of the receptor, which is bound to the cell membrane through constant (C) regions. Adapted from Moss *et al.* (1992).

proliferation. The CD3 complex is physically associated with either CD4 or CD8 receptors depending on the subset of T cell. CD4 determines binding to HLA class II molecules and CD8 to HLA class I (see below).

3.4.2 Antigenic diversity

T and B lymphocytes can specifically recognize a very large range of antigens. This antigenic diversity is based on the variable regions of the T-cell receptor α- and β-chains and immunoglobulin heavy and light chains. These variable regions are the products of two or three different genes, each of which has many different forms. In the T-cell receptor the different gene segments are V D and J for the β-chain and V and J for the α-chain. The approximate number of different forms of each gene segment are listed in *Table 3.3*. As T-cell development occurs in the embryo different combinations of gene segments come together in a process called gene rearrangement to make functional β-chain and α-chain genes that are unique to that particular T cell. An example of the sort of rearrangement that might occur is given in *Figure 3.6*. Further complexity is added by amino acid substitutions during rearrangement. B-cell antibody diversity works in a similar fashion, with different gene segments coming together to make up the variable regions of the light and heavy chains. Nearly 10 million different combinations are possible, each recognizing a different epitope.

Table 3.3: Number of different forms of gene segments in the α- and β-chains of the T-cell antigen receptor (from Moss *et al.*, 1992)

	α-Chain	β-Chain
Variable genes		
V gene segment	50	57
D gene segment	—	2
J gene segment	70	12
Constant genes		
C gene segment	1	2

3.4.3 MHC specificity

T cells can only respond to an antigen if it is presented by another cell expressing specialized receptors called human leukocyte antigens class I or class II. Cytotoxic CD8 + ve T cells interact with HLA class I receptors, and CD4 + ve 'helper' T lymphocytes interact with class II HLA receptors. Class I receptors are expressed on all nucleated cells and present endogenous foreign antigen, that is antigen which is generated within the cell. This generally means viral antigens. Class II receptors are less widely expressed. Constitutively they are expressed by macrophages, dendritic cells and B cells. However, when appropriately stimulated, for example with the cytokine IFN-γ, a large number of cells can express class II receptors, including epithelial cells, fibroblasts and eosinophils.

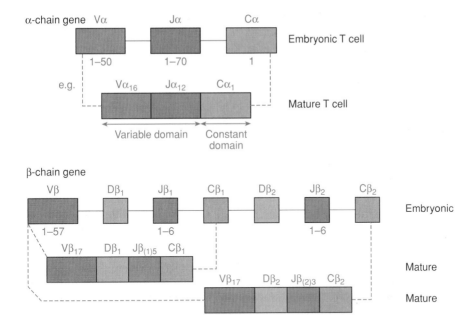

Figure 3.6: An example of gene rearrangement that occurs in T-cell development with combination of variable (V,D), junctional (J) and constant-region (C) genes to produce a functional T-cell receptor gene. Reproduced from Roitt (1991) with permission from Blackwell Scientific Publications Ltd.

The existence of HLA receptors was discovered as a result of organ transplantation studies when it was observed that transplanted donor organs were rejected unless they had the same profile of HLA receptors as the host. They were therefore called antigens of the major histocompatibility complex (MHC). HLA receptors consist of two chains. In the case of class I receptors there is an α-chain of 43 kDa, which combines with an 11-kDa protein called β_2-microglobulin. In the case of the class II receptors there is an α-chain of 34 kDa and a β-chain of 28 kDa.

The structure of the class I molecule has been determined by X-ray crystallography. The α-chain consists of three domains, α_{1-3}. α_3 and β_2-microglobulin are nearest the cell membrane and have a classical immunoglobulin domain structure. The α_1 and α_2 domains form two α-helical ridges on either side of a valley (made up of β-pleated sheets) in which the antigenic peptide being presented is bound (*Figure 3.7*). Analogous to class I structure, it was hypothesized on the basis of sequence homology that the two chains of the class II receptor each have two domains, with α_2/β_2 forming Ig-like domains adjacent to the cell membrane and α_1/β_1 domains forming the peptide-binding structure (*Figure 3.8*). This hypothesis has recently been confirmed with determination of the crystal structure of HLA-DRI.

Like the T-cell antigen receptor, class I and II chains have variable and constant regions. The variable regions are mainly in the groove and ridges,

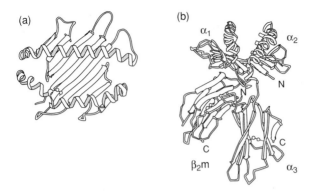

Figure 3.7: Structure of the antigen-binding cleft of HLA class I receptor based on X-ray crystallography. (a) Looking down from the top of the receptor showing the Venus flytrap-like structure of the antigen-binding region. The peptide sits in the floor of the groove which has a β-pleated sheet structure and interacts with the α-helices that make the walls of the groove. (b) Sagittal view of the receptor showing the peptide-binding cleft formed from the α_1 and α_2 domains of the receptor. Reproduced from Bjorkman *et al.* (1987) with permission from Macmillan Magazines Ltd.

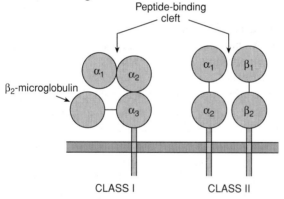

Figure 3.8: Outline of the structure of HLA class I and class II molecules. The class I receptor consists of a three-domain protein chain bound to β_2-micro-globulin and the class II molecule is heterodimeric with each chain having two domains.

which make up the peptide-binding region and the region that binds to the T-cell receptor. Instead of the variability being due to recombination of several distinct genes as with the T-cell receptor, the variability of the HLA receptors is due to polymorphism of the HLA genes, there being many different forms (alleles) of the same gene. Any one individual will only inherit two alleles (one from each parent) of each gene. There are several different class I and class II genes, which are located on chromosome 6 in a region called the major histocompatibility locus. Clustered with the class I and II genes are a number of genes associated with the complement system, proteins involved in cellular transport called heat shock proteins, and the genes for the cytokine tumor necrosis factor (TNF) (*Figure 3.9*). The β_2-microglobulin gene and DRα gene do not vary.

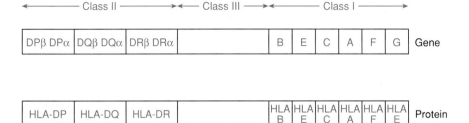

Figure 3.9: The human MHC region on chromosome 6. After Roitt (1991), p. 54, with permission from Blackwell Scientific Publications Ltd.

Different alleles were originally classified by their serological profile, antibodies raised against the MHC receptor being able to distinguish between different alleles. The characterization of an individual's HLA profile by antibodies is the basis of tissue typing. The profile of HLA receptors is called the HLA haplotype. With the advent of rapid techniques for cloning and sequencing the MHC genes it is now possible to compare the serological profile with the exact nucleotide sequence. This has shown even greater polymorphism than suspected from the serological studies. The alleles are given names, for example, *HLA-B27* describes an HLA class I gene at the B locus which is given the arbitrary number B27. As T cells only see antigen when it is presented in conjunction with HLA receptors, the profile of individual HLA receptors is important in determining an individual's response to a given antigen. This is most clearly demonstrated by the links between HLA genes and disease. For example, an individual who expresses an *HLA-B27* gene is at considerably increased risk of developing an inflammatory disease affecting the joints of the spine called ankylosing spondylitis. This may be because there is an increased risk of cross-reactivity between a foreign antigen and a host protein in the joints when presented by the *HLA-B27* receptor. Not only do T cells only 'see' antigen if it is presented by cells expressing class I or class II HLA receptors, but the HLA haplotype of those antigen-presenting cells has to be the same as the HLA haplotype of the T lymphocyte. Thus, cytotoxic T cells from a person with a HLA class I profile of A2 who has recently been infected with influenza will only kill virally infected cells *in vitro* if the infected cells express the A2 HLA class I allele. Similarly, T-cell clones (i.e. a T-cell culture derived from a single T cell so that all the cells have identical antigen receptors and recognize the same antigen) against ovalbumin will only proliferate if the ovalbumin is presented to them by antigen-presenting cells that have the same HLA class II profile as the individual from whom the T cells were cultured. This is called HLA restriction.

3.4.4 Antigen processing

Foreign proteins such as those derived from bacteria have a complex three-dimensional structure. They are not presented whole to the T cell but have to undergo processing in the antigen-presenting cell (APC), where they are broken down into peptide fragments. During antigen processing, foreign antigen is taken into the APC, either by phagocytosis, as is the case with macrophages and dendritic cells, or through internalization of the antigen bound to immunoglobulin receptors, as is the case with B cells. It is then digested within specific vacuoles called lysosomes into peptide fragments that are 15–24 amino acids in length (from a starting protein which may be composed of several hundred amino acids). The fragments are transported to the Golgi apparatus, where they become bound to HLA class II genes during assembly of the α- and β-chains. The HLA class II receptor–antigen complex is then transported to the cell surface, where it is ready to present antigen (*Figure 3.10*). It can be seen that the class II receptor must be able to bind

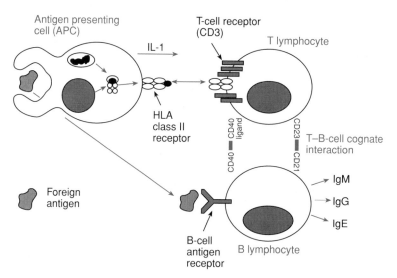

Figure 3.10: Basis of the immune response to foreign antigen. A foreign protein, for example derived from a bacterium, is taken up by an antigen-presenting cell such as a macrophage and digested in lysosomes. Antigenic peptides are bound to HLA class II molecules in the Golgi apparatus, where the HLA class II receptor is assembled, and then transported to the cell surface, where the class II receptor–peptide complex binds to T cells via the T-cell antigen receptor–CD3 complex. This leads to T-cell proliferation and cytokine release. Activated T cells can then interact with B cells, via membrane receptors such as CD40 and CD21/23, to make specific immunoglobulin. B-cells themselves have been stimulated directly by the antigen binding to the B-cell antigen receptor.

a large number of different antigens. This is the case, although different peptide fragments will bind with different avidities. For a given foreign protein the antigenic regions, i.e. those parts of the molecule that trigger an immune response, are determined in part by the avidity with which the various peptide fragments bind to the class II receptors. A single amino acid change in an antigenic peptide can profoundly alter both the avidity with which it binds to the class II receptor and its ability to provoke a T-cell response. Engineering a known antigen, such as a grass pollen, so that it binds more avidly to its class II receptor than the native protein, but does not trigger an immune response, could theoretically be used to block immune responses to specific antigens. This idea will be discussed in more detail in Chapter 7.

3.4.5 Immunoglobulins and the B-cell antigen receptor

B cells produce antibodies, which form the humoral component of the immune system. Antibodies are protein molecules called immunoglobulins, which were the founder members of the immunoglobulin gene superfamily and, like the T-cell receptor, have variable antigen recognition regions and constant regions (*Figure 3.11*). Antibodies are composed of

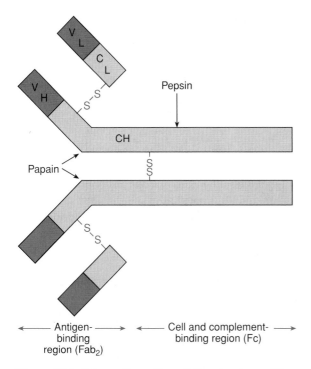

Figure 3.11: Schematic outline of the structure of immunoglobulin. The variable regions (V_H and V_L) of the heavy and light chains are the antigen binding regions whereas the constant region domains of the heavy chains (C_H) bind complement and Fc receptors on leukocytes.

two heavy and two light chains held together by disulfide bonds. Digestion of antibody with papain produces three fragments, two of which are identical and contain the variable regions which bind antigen in a monovalent fashion (Fab; fragment antigen binding), while the third fragment contains the constant region called the Fc (fragment crystallizable), which contains regions for binding complement and cell-binding regions. Leukocyte receptors for immunoglobulin are therefore called Fc receptors. Pepsin cleaves the molecule at a different point to leave the Fc fragment separated from the intact divalent antigen-binding region (Fab_2 fragment). Binding of foreign protein to the antigen recognition region results in triggering of the complement cascade. In addition, binding of antibodies complexed with antigen to Fc receptors on the surface of granulocytes both enhances phagocytosis and causes leukocyte activation.

In humans there are five different types of antibody (isotypes) defined according to differences in the heavy-chain constant region. These are immunoglobulin G (IgG), IgA, IgM, IgE and IgD. In addition there are subgroups within each isotype, for example, four distinct types of IgG (IgG1–4). IgM antibodies are the first to be generated in an immune response, and the B cells producing the antibody then switch from IgM production to generation of the other isotypes (isotype switching). IgG is the main immunoglobulin present in the serum and plays a key role in protection against bacterial infection. IgA is found in high concentrations at mucosal surfaces such as the gut and respiratory tract, and IgE is involved in the host response to parasitic infection as well as allergic disease. The role of IgD, which is a minor isotype, is not clear at present. Antigenic diversity is achieved in the same way as in the T-cell receptor by rearrangement of different genes during B-cell development. Thus, as is the case with T cells, any one B cell produces antibodies with identical antigen recognition elements.

The equivalent of the T-cell receptor on the B cell is an antibody of the IgM type, which is anchored in the membrane by an added hydrophobic region. When a foreign antigen enters the body for the first time it binds to an IgM antibody on the B-cell surface specific for that antigen. This then triggers activation of that B cell which, with T-cell help, proliferates and starts producing large amounts of soluble antibody, identical to the surface receptor antibody, which can then bind the antigen and facilitate its removal. B cells therefore recognize native antigen without any need for processing. They express HLA class II receptors and can present processed antigen to T cells (cognate interaction). Antibody-producing B cells are called plasma cells.

3.4.6 Immunoglobulin E (IgE) synthesis

IgE is of potential importance in asthma both as a marker of atopy and because cross-linking of IgE on mast cells causes the rapid release of a variety of inflammatory mediators. The relationship between asthma and

IgE, although still of uncertain nature, was underlined by a large study of a random population in Tucson, Arizona, that demonstrated a very good correlation between high total IgE levels in the blood (adjusted for age) and the presence of asthma. This was not simply because high IgE was a marker of atopy as there was a better correlation between high IgE and asthma than between atopy and asthma.

A single B cell can produce different immunoglobulin isotypes (i.e. IgM, IgG, IgE) with the same antigen recognition (variable) region. This occurs through splicing (cutting out) the transcribed gene for the constant region of one isotype and inserting the transcribed gene for another. Thus when B cells switch from making IgM to making IgE they stop joining the transcript of the variable VDJ gene to the $C_{H\mu}$ transcript and instead join it to the $C_{H\epsilon}$ transcript (*Figure 3.12*). This is thought to occur by a complex series of regulatory events involving differential activity of various as yet uncharacterized DNA-binding enzymes (recombinases). For B cells to switch to IgE production they need two signals. One of these is the cytokine interleukin 4 (IL-4). The second signal can be provided in several ways, including help from T cells that recognize the same antigen as the B cell or by cross-linking a B-cell receptor called CD40, which is related in structure to the receptors for nerve growth factor and TNF-α. The T-cell signal probably involves either triggering through the CD40 receptor, by interaction with the CD40 ligand on T cells, or binding of a membrane receptor on T cells called CD23 (which is also a low-affinity receptor for IgE) to a membrane receptor on B cells called CD21. Stimulation of B cells through CD21 causes increased production of IgE, and IgE production by B cells can be inhibited by antibodies against CD23. IL-4 alone without a T-cell signal causes the B cell to produce

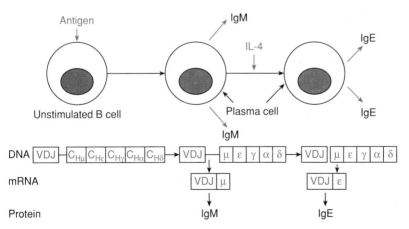

Figure 3.12: Isotype switching on B cells. Antigen initially stimulates the B cell to produce immunoglobulin with a $C_{H\mu}$ constant region (i.e. IgM). Depending on the cytokine signal it receives, the B cell (plasma cell) then switches to producing antibody with the same antigenic specificity (VDJ region) but a different constant region. If the B cell is exposed to IL-4 it will produce IgE ($C_{H\epsilon}$ constant region).

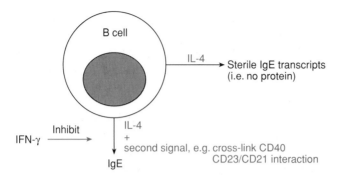

Figure 3.13: Schematic outline of IgE regulation. If a B cell is exposed to IL-4 alone it will produce a sterile IgE transcript that cannot be translated into protein. If IL-4 and an appropriate second signal occurs, such as stimulation via the membrane receptor CD40, mature IgE immunoglobulin is produced. If IFN-γ is present IgE production is inhibited.

sterile $C_{H\varepsilon}$ transcripts, that is they cannot be translated into protein. IFN-γ inhibits IL-4-mediated IgE production in mixed lymphocyte cultures by an as yet undefined mechanism and IL-4 inhibits the production of IFN-γ by lymphocytes (*Figure 3.13*).

3.5 Cell migration

Leukocytes differentiate from uncommitted stem cell precursors in the bone marrow. The development of leukocyte lineages is determined by various growth factors. Some growth factors stimulate the growth of several cells, whereas other growth factors are monospecific. Thus interleukin 3 (IL-3) can stimulate the growth of mast cells, basophils

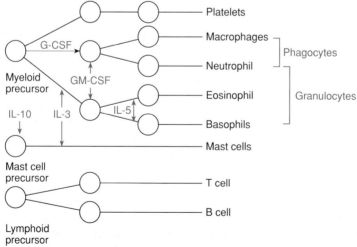

Figure 3.14: Classification of leukocytes with some of the growth factors involved in their development.

and eosinophils, whereas IL-5 can only stimulate the growth and differentiation of eosinophils and possibly basophils (*Figure 3.14*).

As cell types develop from precursors they change morphology: starting as small cells with a single nucleus they gradually take on the appearance of the mature cell type. Most leukocytes when they are mature stop dividing and are released into the blood, but some cell types, for example neutrophils and eosinophils, lose the capacity for further division at this point and are called end-stage cells. Other cells, particularly lymphocytes, can undergo further division. Once released into the blood, leukocytes circulate for a variable period of time before entering the tissues. Some cells constantly recirculate, entering the tissues and then re-entering the blood after a period of time, this being most clearly seen with lymphocytes, which are constantly circulating in search of antigen. Lymphocyte recirculation maximizes the chance of a specific T or B cell coming into contact with the antigen that it recognizes. Thus, lymphocytes home preferentially to the lymph nodes in which they first came into contact with antigen. Lymphocytes from peripheral lymph nodes, such as those in the neck and axillae, will preferentially return to those lymph nodes as opposed to lymph nodes in the gut or lung; alternatively, lymphocytes from the gut or lung will preferentially return to those tissues. This highly regulated process is controlled by specific membrane receptors, called homing receptors, binding to equally specific counter-receptors on endothelium called addressins. These receptors are part of a network of receptors involved in cellular adhesion.

Other cells have less need to recirculate. Neutrophils, whose major role is in the immediate response to tissue injury, need to be able to migrate rapidly from the blood to the site of tissue damage and then neutralize the threat, such as unwelcome bacteria, either by phagocytosis and digestion with intracellular enzymes or by the release of various inflammatory mediators. The neutrophil often dies as a result of this process. Even if it survives, its job is then done and persistence in the tissues risks self-damage from toxic neutrophil-derived mediators. The tissue neutrophil is therefore removed, as part of a process of regulated cell death called apoptosis, by phagocytic macrophages. Macrophages are resident in tissues, where they act as general scavengers engulfing unwanted debris. They are derived mainly from monocytes which have migrated from the blood and differentiated into macrophages in the tissue. Eosinophils are also primarily tissue-dwelling cells with 100–500 tissue eosinophils for every circulating eosinophil. However, they are able to migrate rapidly from the blood into the tissue in certain types of inflammatory response.

It can therefore be seen that the patterns of migration from the blood into tissue differ according to cell function. Migration into tissue occurs in the post-capillary venules as a result of a carefully controlled sequence of events. Initially there is adhesion to the endothelial cell, followed by migration through the vessel wall and then directed locomotion

Receptors   Stages

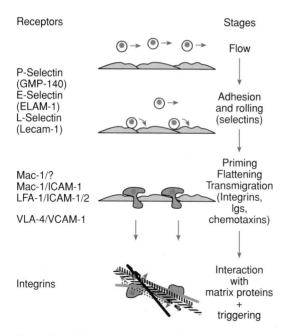

Figure 3.15: Stages involved in leukocyte migration from the blood into the extracellular matrix, and the adhesion receptors involved. Leukocytes initially adhere loosely via selectins and roll along the wall of the blood vessel. After priming, for example by contact with a chemoattractant, they transmigrate using immunoglobulin-like–integrin receptor interactions. Once through the blood vessel wall they bind to extracellular matrix proteins via integrin receptors.

(chemotaxis) under the influence of chemotactic mediators released at the inflammatory focus (*Figure 3.15*). This is most clearly seen with neutrophils shortly after an inflammatory stimulus. These cells, which normally flow unimpeded through the venule, become attached to the endothelial wall and roll slowly along it. The neutrophil then comes to a halt, flattens and starts to crawl through the junctions between endothelial cells (diapedesis). It then dissolves the basement membrane and migrates into the extracellular tissue comprising principally matrix proteins such as fibronectin and fibrinogen.

3.5.1 Adhesion receptors

Like lymphocyte homing, leukocyte migration into tissue is controlled principally by adhesion receptors which are also important in biological functions as diverse as embryogenesis, fertilization of the oocyte with sperm, thrombogenesis and wound healing. There are three main families of adhesion receptors characterized according to structural criteria. The three gene superfamilies are the selectins, the integrins and members of the immunoglobulin gene superfamily (*Figure 3.16*). Adhesion receptors are important in adhesion to endothelium and their ligands are shown in *Table 3.4*.

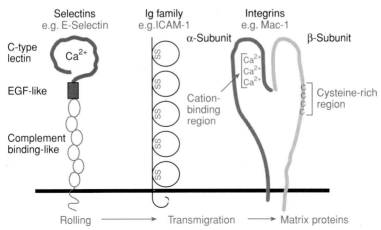

Figure 3.16: Outline of the structure of the major adhesion receptor families involved in leukocyte migration. The selectins have a C-type lectin domain which binds carbohydrate groups on the cell surface. Integrins are two-chain glycoproteins and the immunoglobulin-like receptors possess a number of domains related to members of the immunoglobulin gene superfamily.

Table 3.4: Endothelial/leukocyte adhesion receptors (see Abbreviations, p. ix, for full names)

Endothelium	Gene family	Counter-receptor	Gene family	Leukocyte
ICAM-1	Ig	LFA-1 + Mac-1	Integrin	All leukocytes
ICAM-2	Ig	LFA-1	Integrin	All leukocytes
VCAM-1	Ig	VLA-4	Integrin	All leukocytes except neutrophils
E-selectin	Selectin	Sialyl Lewis X	Carbohydrate	? All leukocytes
P-selectin	Selectin	Sialyl Lewis X	Carbohydrate	? All leukocytes
Glycam-1	Carbohdyrate/ mucin	L-selectin	Selectin	? All leukocytes

There are three members of the selectin family, E-selectin, P-selectin and L-selectin, which are so called because they have an N-terminal domain that is homologous to animal lectins (lectins are proteins that bind sugars). The counter-receptors for selectins are therefore sugars with a defined structure, called sialyl Lewis X. Binding of selectins to their carbohydate ligand is dependent on calcium ions, so they are called calcium-dependent or C-type lectins. The sialyl Lewis X (sLex) sugars are expressed on the cell surface in association with a number of protein and lipid structures. One of these, which is important in lymphoctye homing, is a mucin-like molecule with a structure like a bottle brush, in which a straight rod of protein sticks out from the cell covered in bristle-like O-linked sugars with the sLex structure. This molecule, termed glycam-1, therefore defines a new class of adhesion proteins important in leukocyte migration. Selectins mediate the initial attachment of the cell to the vessel wall and its rolling movement along it.

Integrins form a large family of widely expressed, heterodimeric, glycoprotein membrane receptors. The two protein chains (α and β) which form the receptor are non-covalently (i.e. the association is not through disulfide bonds and is therefore relatively weak) bound at the cell surface. So far about eight β-chains and 13 α-chains have been described, with about 20 receptor pairings identified (*Figure 3.17*). Pairings are restricted. In particular, three β-chains pair with a number of different α-chains to form three subfamilies termed the β_1 (VLA), β_2 (leukocyte) and β_3 integrins. As well as mediating leukocyte binding to endothelium, integrins are important in cell attachment to extracellular matrix proteins.

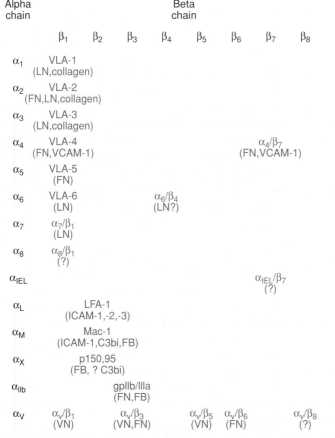

Alpha chain	β_1	β_2	β_3	β_4	β_5	β_6	β_7	β_8
α_1	VLA-1 (LN,collagen)							
α_2	VLA-2 (FN,LN,collagen)							
α_3	VLA-3 (LN,collagen)							
α_4	VLA-4 (FN,VCAM-1)						α_4/β_7 (FN,VCAM-1)	
α_5	VLA-5 (FN)							
α_6	VLA-6 (LN)			α_6/β_4 (LN?)				
α_7	α_7/β_1 (LN)							
α_8	α_8/β_1 (?)							
α_{IEL}							α_{IEL}/β_7 (?)	
α_L		LFA-1 (ICAM-1,-2,-3)						
α_M		Mac-1 (ICAM-1,C3bi,FB)						
α_X		p150,95 (FB, ? C3bi)						
α_{IIb}			gpIIb/IIIa (FN,FB)					
α_V	α_V/β_1 (VN)		α_V/β_3 (VN,FN)		α_V/β_5 (VN)	α_V/β_6 (FN)		α_V/β_8 (?)

Figure 3.17: The integrin receptor family. A number of α- and β-chain associations have been defined with three major subfamilies consisting of the β_1-chain associated with a number of α-chains, the β_2-chain with three α-chains, and the β_3-chain with two α-chains. Most of the receptors are involved in binding to matrix protein with $\alpha_4\beta_1$ and the β_2 integrins involved in leukocyte migration. Ligands are shown in parentheses: FN, fibronectin; FB, fibrinogen; VN, vitronectin; LN, laminin.

The importance of the leukocyte integrins is illustrated by a rare autosomal recessive immunodeficiency disease called leukocyte adhesion deficiency disease (LAD), which is caused by a genetic defect in the β-chain of the leukocyte integrins, resulting in a failure of expression of all three receptors. These patients suffer from severe infections which are often fatal as a result of the inability of the patient's neutrophils, which are highly dependent on the leukocyte integrins, to migrate into the tissues.

The integrins binding to their counter-receptors on the endothelium are responsible for the flattening and transmigration stage of leukocyte migration. Their counter-receptors on endothelium are members of the immunoglobulin superfamily and are therefore related in structure to immunoglobulin molecules and the T-cell receptor. There is a certain selectivity in the use of these receptors by different cell types, and the different patterns of cell migration in both health and inflammation may be partly due to differential use of adhesion receptors. The function of adhesion receptors is controlled either by increasing the numbers of receptors on the cell surface, as is the case with endothelial receptors, or by increasing the affinity of a receptor for its ligand by a structural change in the receptor, usually associated with leukocyte activation. Integrins are regulated in this way. On uninflamed endothelium there is little expression of adhesion receptors so that leukocytes in the blood do not stick and therefore cannot migrate into tissue. However, with the release of inflammatory mediators, adhesion receptors become expressed on the endothelium, making it sticky. *In vitro*, adhesion receptors have different kinetics of up-regulation and are variably expressed. For example, one of the immunoglobulin receptors that may be important in eosinophil adhesion, VCAM-1, is not normally expressed by endothelium but is selectively up-regulated by IL-4, which has little effect on the expression of other endothelial cell adhesion molecules. IL-4 is released in allergic inflammation where eosinophils are predominant cells. It is therefore possible that IL-4/VCAM-1 is responsible for the selective eosinophil accumulation under these circumstances. In support of this hypothesis is the observation that IL-4 transgenic mice (which make large quantities of IL-4) have large numbers of eosinophils in their tissues. Migration from the blood therefore involves a staged process with initial arrest in the venule mediated by selectin receptors, activation by inflammatory mediators and then engagement of the integrin/Ig family receptor pairs, which leads to transmigration. Selective patterns of leukocyte accumulation as seen in different patterns of inflammation may be due to engagement of different sets of adhesion receptors as a result of differential expression.

3.6 Chemoattractants

A fundamental property of leukocytes is the ability to move. This can occur in a random fashion (chemokinesis) or in a directed fashion along a concentration gradient of a chemical mediator to which the cell is responsive (chemotaxis). Chemicals which can cause directed locomotion are called chemoattractants. All chemoattractants stimulate cells, but not all mediators that cause cell activation are chemoattractants, although they usually increase chemokinesis.

A bewildering array of chemicals have been shown to have chemotactic properties *in vitro*. This generally involves the use of a Boyden chamber assay in which cells are separated from the chemical in question by a filter through which the cells have to crawl (*Figure 3.18*). This assay has been criticized for being an *in vitro* phenomenon which has little relevance to *in vivo* mechanisms of migration. However, there is generally a good correlation between the ability of a chemical to promote migration in the Boyden chamber assay and its ability to cause leukocyte accumulation in tissue.

Some cells are better at migrating than others. The neutrophil can move rapidly, in keeping with its role as a rapid response cell, but lymphocytes are less active in the Boyden chamber. This is in agreement with patterns of leukocyte accumulation in acute inflammation, during which the neutrophil is the first cell to arrive followed by the monocyte and then the lymphocyte. Chemoattractants are variable in the degree to which they are selective for cell type. Neutrophils appear to be responsive to a large number of chemicals, whereas other cell types such as the eosinophil are more restricted.

The state of activation is important in determining the responsiveness of a cell to a given chemoattractant. Thus, in general terms, activated cells are more responsive than resting cells, which could be important *in vivo*. For example, when the chemoattractant platelet-activating factor (PAF), which is chemotactic for both eosinophils and neutrophils, was injected into the skin of normal volunteers only neutrophils migrated into the skin. However, injection into the skin of allergic individuals, in whom there is

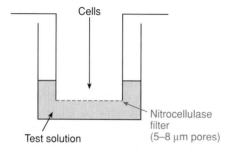

Figure 3.18: The principle of the Boyden chamber. Cells are placed in one well separated from the putative chemoattractants by a filter through which the cells can crawl. After about 1 h the filter is stained and the number of cells which have migrated through the filter counted.

evidence that circulating eosinophils are activated, resulted in the migration of mainly eosinophils into the tissues.

As mentioned above, a large number of chemoattractants have been described. Those with relevance to asthma will be discussed in Chapter 5. Many chemoattractants bind to receptors that share common structural features and are grouped into a gene family. They are characterized by seven membrane-spanning domains and by being G protein linked. G proteins, as described below, are important in cell activation.

3.7 Leukocyte activation and effector function

Leukocytes possess a number of mechanisms for carrying out their role in host defense. These include the antigen-specific activities of T and B cells as well as the non-specific functions of neutrophils, eosinophils and macrophages. The effector functions of leukocytes include locomotion, phagocytosis with subsequent intracellular killing by lysosomal enzymes, and secretion of a variety of chemicals which themselves can have cytotoxic, pro- and anti-inflammatory functions depending upon the circumstances.

Most effector functions are caused by a receptor on the surface of the leukocyte being engaged by its ligand. For example, binding of an immunoglobulin molecule to its Fc receptor on a neutrophil causes both phagocytosis of that immunoglobulin, together with any foreign protein bound to it, as well as triggering the release of various chemical mediators, such as enzymes contained within the neutrophil granule and oxygen radicals generated by a chemical process within the the neutrophil known as the oxygen burst. In normal individuals circulating leukocytes are in a resting state, meaning that their various effector functions are relatively unresponsive to appropriate stimuli. For example, resting neutrophils migrate slowly, phagocytose foreign bodies poorly, and release only small amounts of chemical mediators upon stimulation. This makes teleological sense, for if neutrophils were releasing their mediators in large quantities into the blood this would risk a systemic reaction which would be dangerous to the host. In contrast, leukocytes at inflammatory foci are fully activated cells which are secreting their mediators and are in a highly responsive state for phagocytosis and locomotion. There is also an intermediate state (called 'primed') in which the cell is responsive but not actually degranulating or secreting its mediators (*Figure 3.19*). In effect, there is a continuum between resting and fully activated, rather than the two being distinct states. Chemotactic mediators tend to be effective priming agents but ineffective at promoting secretion, whereas effective secretagogues such as immunoglobulin are not generally chemoattractants.

Engagement of a leukocyte membrane receptor by a priming or activating stimulus starts a series of intracellular events which can result in a range of cellular responses depending on the cell type and nature of the

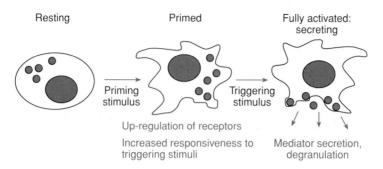

Figure 3.19: Under the influence of priming and triggering stimuli, leukocytes move from a resting to a fully activated state in which they generate and secrete a range of chemical mediators.

stimulus. These include gene activation and new protein synthesis, degranulation, secretion of stored and newly formed mediators, phagocytosis and cellular proliferation. The mechanisms involved in producing these responses are complex and still incompletely understood. The events leading to degranulation of mast cells and the release of histamine after cross-linking of the high-affinity IgE receptor have been studied in some detail and can be used as a model for what are likely to be similar second-messenger events that lead to functional responses in other leukocytes. Cross-linking of the IgE receptor on mast cells results in a number of intracellular events: (i) membrane depolarization; (ii) the influx of extracellular calcium and the release of calcium from intracellular stores; (iii) activation of membrane-bound GTP-binding proteins and turnover of phosphatidylinositol leading to protein kinase activation; (iv) protease activation; (v) changes in intracellular concentrations of cyclic AMP.

3.7.1 Role of calcium in cell activation

Extracellular calcium is required for optimal release of histamine from IgE-triggered mast cells. There is little histamine release in calcium-free medium, calcium chelating agents such as EDTA inhibit most of the histamine release and calcium ionophores (agents that force calcium into cells), such as A23187, causing maximal histamine release. Normal extracellular concentrations of calcium are 1 mM compared with 0.1 mM intracellularly. Injection of calcium into mast cells results in degranulation. Ions of the rare earth lanthanum, which block membrane calcium channels, inhibit histamine release. It seems therefore that cross-linking of IgE receptors causes membrane depolarization within 1 min followed by increased permeability of membrane calcium channels, allowing calcium influx into the cell, which is optimal within 5 min. Unregulated entry of calcium into the cell, as in the case of stimulation with a calcium ionophore, causes 100% histamine release but leads to cell death. Receptor cross-linking causes suboptimal release but does not result in cell death. This is because receptor cross-linking results in only a transient increase in membrane permeability for calcium. Cross-linking of mast cells in a calcium-free medium, causes desensitization in that they become refractory to a second antigen stimulus in the presence of calcium. This is probably due to a transient loss of the ability of receptor cross-linking to cause calcium permeability as the cells can still be triggered by calcium ionophore.

3.7.2 Phosphatidylinositol turnover

Phosphatidylinositol (PI) is a membrane phospholipid that is the starting point in a second-messenger pathway. Through addition of phosphate groups by ATP-dependent kinases, it becomes firstly a PI-4 monophosphate (PIP), then a PI-4,5-biphosphate (PIP_2), which is a substrate for phospholipase C, which in turn has been activated by a receptor-bound GTP-binding protein. Phospholipase C converts PIP_2 into inositol-1,4,5-triphosphate (IP_3) and diacyglycerol (DAG). IP_3 results in release of calcium from intracellular stores, and DAG causes activation of protein kinase C, a 77-kDa protein that catalyzes the phosphorylation of serine and threonine residues in a large number of proteins. Phorbol esters directly activate protein kinase C. At the end of the pathway, IP_3 and DAG can be recycled back to PI (*Figure 3.20*).

3.7.3 Cyclic nucleotides

A second important intracellular signaling pathway is adenylate cyclase/cyclic AMP (*Figure 3.21*). It was observed that β-agonists (drugs that activate the β-adrenoreceptor) inhibit histamine release from mast cells. Activation of the G protein-linked β-adrenoreceptor causes activation of adenylate cyclase, which transforms ATP into cyclic AMP, which in turn activates protein kinase A, which catalyzes phosphorylation of serine residues. Other drugs that increase levels of cyclic AMP, for example theophylline, which inhibits the action of phosphodiesterase, also inhibit mast cell degranulation.

3.7.4 GTP-binding proteins

Many membrane receptors involved in cell activation are coupled in the membrane to proteins that bind GDP and GTP (G proteins). In the resting state these G proteins exist as a trimer with α-, β- and γ-chains. The α-chain binds to GDP, which stabilizes the complex. Engagement of the membrane receptor by its ligand results in the GDP being replaced by GTP, which causes dissociation of the subunits of the G protein. The α-chain–GTP complex is able to activate a number of intracellular proteins,

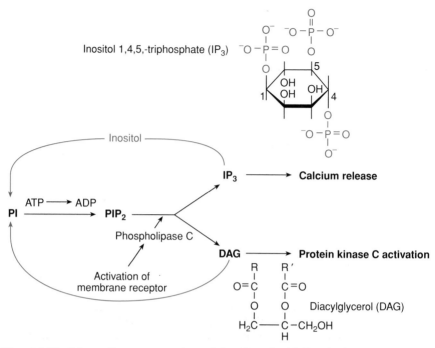

Figure 3.20: Schematic representation of the phosphatidylinositol (PI) second-messenger pathway. PI in the cell membrane is phosphorylated to phosphatidylinositol-4,5-biphosphate, which is hydrolyzed by the membrane-bound enzyme phospholipase C, which has been activated by a ligand binding to its membrane receptor. This results in the generation of diacylglycerol (DAG) and inositol-1,4,5-triphosphate (IP_3), whose structures are shown. DAG leads to activation of protein kinase C and IP_3 to release of calcium from intracellular stores. DAG and IP_3 can be recycled back to resynthesize PI.

which leads to transmission of the signal into the cell (*Figure 3.22*). This appears to be a general method for transducing signals: for example there are G proteins for activation of phospholipase C, distinct from G proteins involved in regulating the adenylate cyclase system of G proteins and G proteins involved in degranulation. Two families of GTP-binding proteins can be distinguished by the inhibitory effects of either pertussis or cholera toxin. There is both a G protein (G_s) that stimulates adenylate cyclase, and a G protein (G_i) that inhibits its activity. G_i is inhibited by pertussis toxin and G_s by cholera toxin.

3.7.5 Protein phosphorylation

Changes in the phosphorylation state are important in changing the energy state and therefore the function of a protein. Intracellular ATP is required for histamine secretion and histamine secretion is dependent on glycolysis and to a lesser extent oxidative phosphorylation to supply ATP

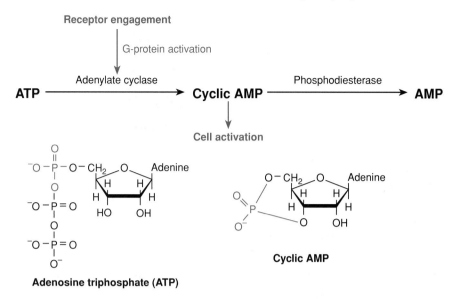

Figure 3.21: The adenylate cyclase/cyclic AMP second-messenger system involves the generation of cAMP from ATP, a process catalyzed by the membrane-bound enzyme adenylate cyclase, which is activated as a result of a ligand engaging with a membrane receptor, leading to G-protein activation. Increased levels of cAMP result in a number of cellular events mediated by activation of protein kinase A. cAMP is degraded to AMP by the action of phosphodiesterase, an enzyme inhibited by theophylline, a drug widely used as a bronchodilator in the treatment of asthma.

to the cell. Cell activation results in the transient phosphorylation of many proteins as well as the dephosphorylation of constitutively phosphorylated proteins by phosphatase. Many receptors, particularly growth factor receptors, are enzymes with tyrosine kinase activity in their cytoplasmic regions, which is activated when ligand binding occurs.

3.7.6 Exocytosis

Whatever the intermediate events, one of the final stages in mediator release from mast cells and granulocytes is fusion of the granule with the cell membrane and release of the granule contents, a process called exocytosis. This appears to be a stepwise process in which individual granules fuse with the cell membrane, releasing their contents into the extracellular environment. Alternatively, cells can release their granule contents through a process called piecemeal degranulation, in which granule contents are transported from granule to cell membrane by vesicles that bud from granules and traverse the cytoplasm. This gives rise to empty non-fused cytoplasmic granules that can be readily identified in tissue sections, particularly in eosinophils.

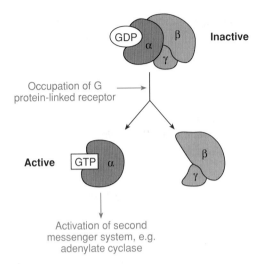

Figure 3.22: Guanyl nucleotide-binding proteins (G proteins) are linked to a number of membrane receptors which have a characteristic seven-transmembrane domain structure. Activation of G proteins is the first step in many second-messenger events. G proteins are a family of proteins with the common structure of an α-, β- and γ-chain, which in the inactive state are complexed with the α-chain bound to GDP. Receptor–ligand binding results in the exchange of GDP for GTP, which causes dissociation of the α-chain from the β- and γ-chains. The α-chain–GTP complex is in the active state, and can activate other components of the second-messenger cascade, such as adenylate cyclase and phospholipase.

3.8. Summary

The inflammatory process is an integral part of the host response to insult and is designed to protect the host against pathogens that threaten its integrity. It has an innate component and an adaptive component, which responds specifically to individual insults through recognition of specific antigen by T and B lymphocytes. Triggering of these cells leads to a series of events which involves interaction with other leukocytes as well as cells resident in tissues, such as mast cells and macrophages, together with the generation of a complex array of mediators. The cells and mediators that play major roles in the inflammatory process integral to asthma are described in the next two chapters.

Further reading

General reading

Corrigan, C.J. and Kay, A.B. (1992) Lymphocytes in allergy and asthma. in *Allergy* (Holgate, S.T. and Church, M.K., Eds). Gower, London.

Roitt, I. (1991) *Essential Immunology*, 7th Edn. Blackwell Scientific Publications, Oxford.

Whaley, K. and Burt, A.D. (1992) Inflammation, healing and repair. in *Muir's Textbook of Pathology*, 13th Edn (MacSween, R.N.M. and Whaley, K., Eds). Edward Arnold, London, pp. 112–165.

T-cell antigen recognition

Moss, P.A.H., Rosenberg, W.M.C. and Bell, J.I. (1992) The human T-cell receptor in health and disease. *Annu. Rev. Immunol.,* **10,** 71–96.

Steinman, R.M. (1991) The dendritic cell system and its role in immunogenicity. *Annu. Rev. Immunol.,* **9,** 271–296.

Unanue, E. (1984) Antigen presenting function of the macrophage. *Annu. Rev. Immunol.,* **2,** 395–428.

IgE regulation

Armitage, R.J., MacDuff, B.M., Anderson, D.M. *et al.* (1992) Molecular and biological characterization of a murine ligand for CD40. *Nature,* **357,** 80.

Geha, R.S. (1992) Regulation of IgE synthesis in humans. *J. Allergy Clin. Immunol.,* **90,** 143–150.

Maggi, E., Parronchi, P., Manetti, R., Simonelli, C., Piccini, M.-P., Rugiu, F.S., Carli, M., Ricci, M. and Romagnani, S. (1992) Reciprocal regulatory effects of IFN-γ and IL-4 on the *in vitro* development of human Th1 and Th2 clones. *J. Immunol.,* **148,** 2142–2147.

Vercelli, D., Jabara, H.H., Lauener, R.P. and Geha, R.S. (1990) Interleukin-4 inhibits the synthesis of interferon-γ and induces the synthesis of IgE in mixed lymphocyte cultures. *J. Immunol.,* **144,** 570.

Adhesion receptors

Butcher, E.C. (1990) Cellular and molecular mechanisms that direct leukocyte traffic. *Am. J. Pathol.,* **136,** 3–11.

Butcher, E.C. (1991) Leukocyte–endothelial cell recognition: Three (or more) steps to specificity and diversity. *Cell,* **67,** 1033–1036.

Harlan, J.M. and Liu, E. (Eds) (1992) *Adhesion: Its Role in Inflammatory Diseases.* W.H. Freeman & Co., New York.

Lasky, L.A., Singer, M.S., Dowbenico, D. *et al.* (1992) An endothelial ligand for L-selectin is a novel mucin-like molecule. *Cell,* **69,** 927–938.

Springer, T.A. (1990) Adhesion receptors of the immune system. *Nature,* **346,** 425–434.

Springer, T.A. and Lasky, L.A. (1991) Sticky sugars for selectins. *Nature,* **349,** 196–197.

Zimmerman, G.A., Prescott, S.M. and McIntyre, T. (1992) Endothelial interactions with granulocytes: tethering and signalling molecules. *Immunol. Today,* **13,** 93–100.

The human major histocompatibility complex and HLA receptors

Bjorkman, P.J., Saper, M.A., Samraoui, B., Bennett, W.S., Stromager, J.L. and Wiley, D.C. (1987) Structure of the human class 1 histocompatibility antigen HLA-A2. *Nature,* **329,** 506-512.

Brown, J.H., Jardetzky, T.S., Gorga, J.C., Stern, L.J., Urban, R.G., Stromager, J.L. and Wiley, D.C. (1993) Three-dimensional structure of the human class II histocompatibility antigen HLA-DR1. *Nature,* **364,** 33–39.

Charron, D. (1990) Molecular basis of human leukocyte antigen class II disease associations. *Adv. Immunol.,* **48,** 107–159.

Marsh, S.G.E. and Bodmer, J.G. (1989) HLA-DR and DQ epitopes and monoclonal antibody specificity. *Immunol. Today,* **10**, 305.tsave

Trowsdale, J., Ragoussis, J. and Campbell, R.D. (1991) Map of the human MHC. *Immunol. Today,* **12,** 443–446.

Leukocyte activation

Karin, M. (1992) Signal transduction from cell surface to nucleus in development and disease. *FASEB J.,* **6,** 2581–2590.

Chapter 4

Inflammation in asthma II.
The cells

4.1 Introduction

Our understanding of the role of resident and migratory cells in the bronchial mucosa in the pathogenesis of asthma comes from two main sources: clinical studies, which have defined the pathological differences between asthmatic and normal tissue, and *in vitro* studies that have investigated the extent to which inflammatory mediators derived from various cell types could cause the tissue damage characteristic of asthma. Current evidence suggests that certain cell types play a primary role in the pathogenesis of asthma, whereas other cells have a more subsidiary function. Primary effector cells include eosinophils, mast cells and T lymphocytes, whereas secondary cells include neutrophils, macrophages and epithelial cells. This chapter discusses in more detail the characteristics of these cells and the roles they are thought to play in asthma.

4.2 Primary effector cells

4.2.1 The T lymphocyte

As discussed in Chapter 1, there is good clinical evidence, particularly in atopic asthmatics and occupational asthma, that at least the initiating event in asthma is exposure to inhaled antigen to which the individual has become sensitized. This immediately suggests a role for T and B lymphocytes, as these are the only cells capable of recognizing antigen in a specific fashion. T cells are derived from the bone marrow and during fetal development pass through the thymus, where they mature. At this point T cells that recognize self antigen are removed. Mature T cells which emerge from the thymus are divided into a number of subsets according to the expression of various cell surface receptors.

T-cell subsets. One important division is between CD4 + ve and CD8 + ve cells. CD4 + ve cells are generally involved in cytokine production and assisting B cells to make antibody. They are therefore called helper or inducer cells. CD8 + ve cells have a cytotoxic role and are involved in host protection against viral infections. Because of their cytotoxic role they appeared to suppress antibody production and were at one time called suppressor cells. Whether T cells that truly suppress immune functions exist is still not clear.

T cells can be further subdivided according to the cytokine mediators which they generate when stimulated. This was first described in the mouse. Using special culture techniques it is possible to obtain antigen-reactive T cells which are monoclonal, that is they share identical T-cell receptors (these are called clonal T cells or T-cell clones). It was observed that mouse T-cell clones when stimulated with antigen could be categorized according to which cytokine they secreted. One type secreted IL-2 and IFN-γ and another type secreted IL-4, IL-5 and IL-10. Both types secreted IL-3 and GM-CSF. Some T-cell clones secreted a mixture of cytokines. These types of T cell were called, respectively, Th1, Th2 and Th0. Which T-cell clones were generated depended on the type of antigen, the strain of mouse and the culture conditions. This had immediate implications for asthma because IL-5 is an important and selective hematopoietic factor for eosinophils and IL-4 results in isotype switching of B cells to the generation of IgE. Furthermore, it was observed that IFN-γ suppressed the generation of Th2 cells and IL-4 suppressed the production of Th1 cells.

At first, human T-cell clones did not appear to fall into such neat subdivisions, with most T-cell clones producing a mixture of cytokines. However, more recently it has been possible to generate Th1- and Th2-type clones from humans. For example, house dust mite (HDM)-specific T-cell clones from atopic individuals sensitized to HDM allergen were Th2 in type, whereas HDM T-cell clones from non-atopic subjects were Th1 in type. Moreover, *in situ* hybridization studies demonstrated that IL-4 and IL-5 mRNA was generated in the skin of atopic individuals after allergen challenge (a model of allergic inflammation), whereas IL-2 and IFN-γ transcripts were generated during the tuberculin reaction to mycobacterial antigens (a classic Th1 type of reaction). This work has been confirmed in the nasal mucosa after allergen challenge. Similarly, in both clinical asthma and after allergen challenge to the lung IL-4 and IL-5 mRNA was expressed by T cells in BAL fluid and endobronchial biopsies. There is therefore good evidence that in atopic asthmatics a Th2-type response is occurring in the airways. The situation in intrinsic asthma has not been as well described. However, there is increasing evidence that intrinsic asthma is associated with increased amounts of IL-5 without any increase in IL-4 production. Thus, increased amounts of IL-5, but not IL-4, have been found in the peripheral blood and BAL fluid from non-atopic asthmatics, and increased expression of mRNA for IL-5 but not IL-4 has been observed in peripheral blood mononuclear cells from non-atopic asthmatics. This raises the possibility that intrinsic asthma is associated with activation of a novel type of T lymphocyte subset that secretes IL-5 but not IL-4.

The underlying mechanism by which T cells become Th1 or Th2 type is not clear. A number of factors appear to play a part, including the nature of the antigen (metazoan parasitic antigens appear to be particularly good at inducing a Th2 type of response), the route of antigen administration, and the dose of antigen. The fact that patients infected with helminthic parasites invariably have an eosinophilia suggests that most people can develop a Th2-type response to some antigens. It is likely that the atopic state is due to a genetically determined propensity to develop a Th2-type response to allergens.

The existence of a genetic component is supported by experiments in related strains of mice. Balb/c mice develop a Th2-type response characterized by high IgE levels and an eosinophilia when infected with the parasite *Leishmonia major*, whereas a related strain develops a Th1-type response. Interestingly, in this case the Th1 type of response is more protective against infection. In addition, administration of the Balb/c mice with IFN-γ resulted in switching to a Th1 type of response, an observation with therapeutic potential in asthma. Interestingly, the administration of high-dose glucocorticoids to asthmatics resulted in a relative switching from the generation of the mRNA for cytokines IL-4 and IL-5 in the airways to IL-2 and IFN-γ. This was associated with an improvement in asthma and a fall in the number of eosinophils in the airways. Whether this was due to individual T cells switching from a Th2 to a Th1 type of cytokine generation or differential suppression of Th2 over Th1 cells is not clear. Indeed, the extent to which individual T cells are fixed in their pattern of cytokine generation is at present not fully understood. Nevertheless, it can be seen that the idea of differential secretion of cytokines by subsets of T cells in response to different antigens is likely to be of central importance in asthma. In support of this possibility is a recent observation that IFN-α, when given to allergen-challenged mice, prevents an airways eosinophilia, possibly through blocking activation of Th2 lymphocytes.

T-cell activation. A second important T-cell subdivision is between naive and memory cells. T cells are first presented with antigen in the lymph nodes, where they proliferate to form lymphoblasts which are fully activated and a pool of primed cells which are much more responsive to antigen than naive cells. For example, naive cells have very precise requirements for antigen presentation whereas primed T cells can recognize antigen presented by a wide range of cells bearing MHC class II molecules. This pool of primed or memory cells then recirculates through the blood and lymphatic tissue ready for a rapid response to a further antigenic stimulus. Memory to antigen persists for many years. As discussed in the previous chapter, lymphocytes do not recirculate randomly but preferentially home to the lymphatic tissue and organ in which they first encountered antigen.

Naive and memory cells can be readily distinguished by distinct profiles of membrane receptor expression. In particular, they express different isotypes of a receptor expressed by all leukocytes called CD45. Naive T cells express the CD45RO form and memory cells the CD45RA form. In the lungs most T cells appear to be memory cells, consistent with the lung being a major organ of antigen entry. The biochemical basis of the memory phenotype is not known. Recent studies have suggested that over time CD45RA + ve memory cells return to being CD45RO + ve, suggesting that the memory phenotype is a long-lasting activation phenotype.

T cells and asthma. Evidence that T cells have a major role in the pathogenesis of asthma is provided by a number of studies. T cells, when stimulated with antigen, express a number of receptors not expressed by resting cells. These 'activation' receptors can be used as markers of T-cell activation. They include CD25, CD28, CD69 and the VLA-1 adhesion receptor. CD69 is expressed very early in T-cell activation, whereas VLA-1 is expressed very late. In acute severe asthma there are increased numbers of CD25 + ve (i.e. activated) CD4 + ve T cells in the blood, which return to normal levels on treatment. As discussed in Chapter 2 there are increased numbers of CD25 + ve T cells in the airways of intrinsic, extrinsic and occupational asthmatics as well as patients who have died from asthma. Corticosteroids are particularly effective at blocking T-cell activation. T cells are intimately associated with eosinophil accumulation in tissues, and IL-4 production by Th2 lymphocytes could be responsible for the production of specific IgE by B cells in atopic asthmatics.

The exact role of the activated T cells in asthmatic airways is still not known. One possibility is that on inhalation of an allergen such as HDM, to which the person is atopic specific Th2-type T cells are recruited into the bronchi, where they start producing IL-5 and IL-4. However, it appears that only a relatively small proportion of T cells at sites of allergen challenge in the skin are antigen specific, although this is a higher proportion than found in the peripheral blood. This modest concentration of allergen-specific T cells could be due to local proliferation or selective recruitment. Nevertheless, many of the T cells appear to be have been recruited non-specifically, possibly under the influence of locally generated T-cell chemotactic agents. This is consistent with findings in other inflammatory diseases, in which analysis of the antigen receptor on T cells isolated from inflammatory lesions has shown less evidence of oligoclonality than would be expected if the T cells were all reacting to a single antigen. Another alternative is that allergen-specific Th2 cells are activated in the lymph nodes and that IL-5 and IL-4 so generated increase the number of eosinophils released from the bone marrow, with more local factors being responsible for the selective accumulation of eosinophils in the lung. Understanding the exact role of T cells will therefore require a greater understanding of their pattern of migration into the lung in asthma.

In summary, activated Th2 cells are found in the airways of asthmatics but not normal controls. IL-5 secreted by these T cells may be responsible for the recruitment of eosinophils into the lung and IL-4 for the generation of specific IgE by B cells in the airways and local lymph nodes.

4.2.2 Eosinophils

As discussed in Chapter 2, the most striking and consistent difference between asthmatic and normal airways is the presence of increased numbers of activated eosinophils in asthma. This, together with the realization that eosinophils can release large amounts of potent inflammatory mediators which could cause the pathological changes characteristic of asthma, has led to a current consensus that eosinophil-derived mediators are a likely primary cause of asthma (*Figure 4.1*). The biology of this cell will therefore be discussed in some detail.

Eosinophil structure and membrane receptors. Eosinophils are character-ized by a bilobed nucleus and characteristic large granules which are round or ovoid in shape and often have an electron-dense core (*Figure 4.2*). The granules are made up mainly of four proteins which, because they contain large amounts of basic amino acids such as arginine, are strongly negative, with pI values in the region of 10. As a result they bind avidly to acidic dyes such as eosin, which is how they got their name over 100 years ago when first described by Ehrlich. The four proteins, called major basic protein (MBP), eosinophil cationic protein (ECP), eosinophil peroxidase (EPO) and eosinophil-derived neurotoxin (EDN), are all toxic to mammalian cells, including bronchial epithelium. They are also toxic for helminthic parasites, supporting the idea that the teleological role for eosinophils is to protect against certain forms of parasite infection. These proteins are discussed in detail in Chapter 5.

Eosinophil receptors. Like all leukocytes, eosinophils express a large number of membrane receptors. These include adhesion receptors, Fc receptors, which bind immunoglobulin and are involved in triggering secretion, receptors for soluble mediators and receptors such as CD69, of unknown function (*Figure 4.3*). The receptor profile of eosinophils is distinct from that of other cells, although no completely specific eosinophil receptors have been described. Many receptors are constitu-tively expressed, although their level of expression can change with the activation state of the cell. In addition, cell stimulation, particularly with cytokines, results in the synthesis and expression of receptors not normally seen on resting eosinophils (*Table 4.1*). Some of these newly

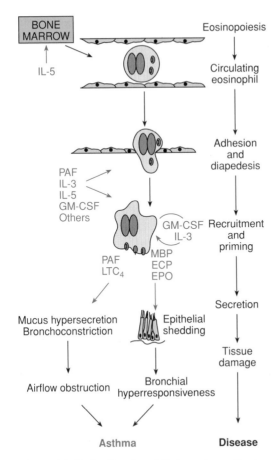

Figure 4.1: Role of eosinophils in asthma. Eosinophils differentiate from precursor cells in the bone marrow under the influence of growth factors, particularly IL-5. They then migrate from the peripheral blood to the airways of asthmatics, during which process they become activated and secrete a number of mediators which could potentially cause the pathological changes characteristic of asthma.

expressed receptors, such as CD69, which are expressed by eosinophils in asthmatic airways but not on eosinophils in the peripheral blood, may be important in triggering the cell to release its mediators.

Eosinopoiesis. Eosinophils are end-stage cells (i.e. they do not undergo further cell division) derived from stem cell precursors in the bone marrow under the influence of various growth factors. IL-3, IL-5 and GM-CSF have growth activity for eosinophils, with only IL-5 being specific (although it may also have growth activity for basophils). An increase in the number of eosinophils in the blood is not usually associated with increased numbers of other cell types, suggesting that a highly eosinophil-specific growth factor is involved in causing a blood eosinophilia. Evi-

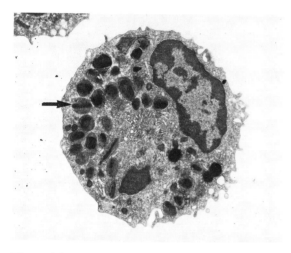

Figure 4.2: Transmission electron micrograph of an eosinophil showing the characteristic specific granules with electron-dense central cores (arrow). × 7000. Courtesy of Dr Ann Dewar, National Heart and Lung Institute, London.

dence that this is IL-5 comes from transgenic mice, in which the IL-5 gene has been genetically engineered to cause overproduction. These mice have a marked eosinophilia without any increase in other cell types. Interestingly, these mice are perfectly healthy, suggesting that more than

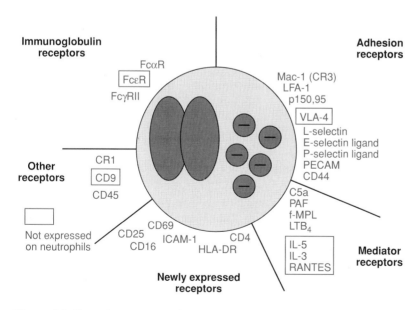

Figure 4.3: Some important eosinophil membrane receptors involved in adhesion and responses to soluble mediators, Fc receptors involved in triggering of eosinophil secretion, and newly expressed receptors induced as part of the process of eosinophil activation.

Table 4.1: Eosinophil receptors whose expression is altered by the activation state of the cell

Receptor	Expression on peripheral blood eosinophils	Expression after culture with IL-3 *in vitro*	Expression on tissue eosinophils (e.g. BAL eosinophils) in asthma
CR3 (Mac-1)	+ +	+ + +	+ + +
CD4	+ / −	+	+ / −
CD25	−	+	+ / −
HLA-DR	+ / −	+	+
ICAM-1	−	+ / −	+ / −
λ-selectin	+	Not reported	−
CD16	−	+ (IFN-γ not IL-3)	−
CD69	−	+	+

simply a high eosinophil count is required to cause tissue damage. The various stages of eosinophil differentiation can be seen morphologically with the gradual development of the characteristic eosinophil granules and bilobed nucleus (*Figure 4.4*). Eosinophils are developmentally most closely related to basophils.

Eosinophil migration. The question of how eosinophils get from the bloodstream into the airways in asthma is of great importance, as selective blockage of eosinophil accumulation in the airways may have considerable therapeutic potential in asthma. Three possible mechanisms have been advanced to explain the accumulation of eosinophils without

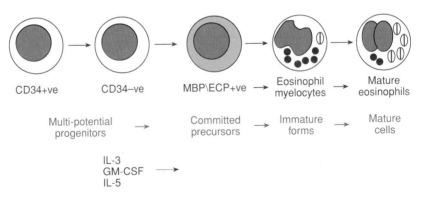

Figure 4.4: Schematic representation of the stages in eosinophil differentiation. Uncommitted stem cells stop expressing the differentiation receptor CD34 and then differentiate towards mature eosinophils under the influence of cytokine growth factors. Initially eosinophil precursors have homogeneous cytoplasm but stain for granule proteins. At the myelocyte stage, specific core-containing granules can be seen, but these are few in number and are interspersed amongst homogeneous granules. Mature eosinophils have bilobed nuclei and many specific granules, as well as lipid bodies and primary granules.

increased numbers of neutrophils, in the airways in asthma: a selective adhesion pathway; an eosinophil-specific chemoattractant; and prolonged survival in the airways under the influence of eosinophil-active cytokines.

Eosinophil adhesion. In most respects eosinophil expression of adhesion receptors is similar to that of neutrophils. However, evidence that eosinophils may be able to use alternative adhesion pathways to neutrophils comes from patients with leukocyte adhesion deficiency disease (LAD). In some of these patients eosinophils, but not neutrophils, could be seen in the extracellular tissues, suggesting that eosinophils do not rely solely on the leukocyte integrins to pass through the endothelium. The likely reason for this is that eosinophils, unlike neutrophils, express the integrin receptor VLA-4 and as a result can bind VCAM-1 on the endothelium. This observation is of particular interest because IL-4, as well as promoting IgE synthesis, is able to up-regulate the expression of VCAM-1 on endothelial cells in culture without affecting the expression of other endothelial adhesion molecules. It has now been shown that IL-4 is able to enhance the adhesion and transmigration of eosinophils through cultured endothelial cells by a VLA-4/VCAM-1-dependent adhesion pathway, but has no effect on neutrophils. Interestingly, IL-4 transgenic mice have eosinophils in their tissues, and there is also some evidence that the expression of VCAM-1 is up-regulated on the endothelium of the bronchial vessels after allergen challenge. Further support for the importance of VLA-4 in eosinophil adhesion in asthma is provided by a study in which anti-VLA-4 mAb inhibited the migration of eosinophils into guinea-pig skin, caused by either chemotactic mediators or immunological challenge. These studies therefore suggest that VLA-4/VCAM-1 interactions may be partly responsible for the selective migration of eosinophils into the lung in asthma. However, expression of VCAM-1 on bronchial endothelium in clinical asthma is weak or non-existent, which rather confounds the *in vitro* and animal evidence. The importance of VLA-4 and VCAM-1 in eosinophil adhesion in asthma is therefore unclear at the moment.

Another group of studies on monkeys who have a natural sensitivity to ascaris worm have emphasized the importance of ICAM-1 in eosinophil accumulation. These monkeys, when chronically challenged with ascaris antigen by inhalation, develop an airways eosinophilia and bronchial hyperresponsiveness. Both the eosinophilia and the BHR can be inhibited by an antibody against ICAM-1. These important experiments are discussed further in Chapter 7. Our current understanding of adhesion receptors involved in eosinophil migration is summarized in *Table 4.2*.

Adhesion receptors are not just involved in migration through the endothelium. They also interact with the matrix proteins in the extracellular tissue, for example VLA-4 is a receptor for fibronectin, and they are undoubtedly important in eosinophil interaction with the bronchial epithelium. The asthmatic epithelium, unlike normal epithe-

Table 4.2: Eosinophil adhesion receptors and their counter-structures

Eosinophil receptor	Endothelial receptor	Matrix protein
Integrin		
VLA-4 ($\alpha_4\beta_1$)	VCAM-1	Fibronectin
VLA-6 ($\alpha_6\beta_1$)		Laminin
LFA-1	ICAM-1, ICAM-2	
Mac-1	ICAM-1	Fibrinogen
Immunoglobulin-like		
PECAM	PECAM	
Selectin		
L-selectin	Glycam-1	
Carbohydrate		
P-selectin ligand	P-selectin	
E-selectin ligand	E-selectin	

lium, expresses ICAM-1. It is therefore possible that eosinophil-mediated epithelial damage is due in part to eosinophils being able to bind to epithelial cells through LFA-1–ICAM-1 interactions.

In both steady-state asthmatics and normal subjects there is considerable expression of both E-selectin and ICAM-1 on the bronchial vascular endothelium with only minor increases in asthmatics. Thus, if adhesion receptors are seen as a gate through which leukocytes must pass before entering the tissues, in the airways that gate seems to be permanently open to all leukocytes. There is therefore little evidence at the moment for a selective adhesion pathway being important in regulating eosinophil migration into the airways in asthma.

Eosinophil chemoattractants. An attractive idea is that eosinophil accumulation is due to the effect of a chemotactic mediator which is selective for eosinophils. A large number of eosinophil chemoattractants have been described, generally using the Boyden chamber system, with some conflicting evidence as to their effectiveness (*Table 4.3*). Most selective chemoattractants identified to date are weak, whereas most effective mediators are non-selective. It is possible that a combination of a weak but selective agent such as IL-5 is working in concert with suboptimal concentrations of a strong but non-selective agent such as PAF. In addition, it is possible that the *in vitro* Boyden assay is misleading. For example, IL-5 is a weak chemotactic factor *in vitro*, but when anti-IL-5 antibodies are given to guinea pigs the eosinophil accumulation seen in the airways after allergen challenge is decreased. This is a rapid effect and could not be due to inhibition of eosinopoiesis. Furthermore, after allergen challenge in the nose in humans there was a very good correlation between expression of mRNA for IL-5 as detected by *in situ* hybridization and the number of eosinophils. IL-5 may therefore be the mediator responsible for eosinophil accumulation although the exact mechanisms whereby this might occur is not clear. It has recently been described that RANTES, a chemotactic peptide related to IL-8 and

Table 4.3: Eosinophil chemotactic factors

Chemoattractant	Activity	Selectivity
Lipids		
PAF	High	No
LTB4	Moderate	No
8s,15s,di-HETE	Moderate	No
Low molecular weight peptides		
C5a	High	No
f-MLP	Weak	No
ECF-a tetrapeptides	Negligible	—
Cytokines		
IL-5	Weak	Yes
IL-3	Weak	Yes
GM-CSF	Weak	No
RANTES	High	Yes
IL-8	Weak	No

IL-5, IL-3 and GM-CSF are only active on eosinophils from normal donors.

released by T cells and monocytes, is chemotactic for eosinophils but not neutrophils. This is therefore a candidate chemoattractant for eosinophils, although whether it is released in asthmatic airways is not known.

Eosinophil survival. Eosinophils normally undergo apoptosis and die in culture after a few days. However, if they are cultured in the presence of a number of cytokines such as IL-5, IL-3 and GM-CSF their survival is prolonged by up to several weeks. Cytokine-induced eosinophil survival is inhibited by corticosteroids. These and other eosinophil-active cytokines are released in asthmatic airways and may therefore be responsible for eosinophil accumulation through prolonging their persistence in tissues. Eosinophils cultured on fibronectin generate GM-CSF and IL-3, which results in their own autocrine-induced survival. Interaction with matrix proteins, particularly fibronectin, may therefore be very important in determining the tissue localization of eosinophils.

Eosinophil mediators and secretory triggers. As mentioned above, eosinophils can generate an array of potent pro-inflammatory mediators. These can be divided into three groups: those preformed and stored in the eosinophil granules; those newly derived from membrane phospholipids; and cytokines secreted as a result of protein synthesis (*Figure 4.5*). Whether an activated eosinophil generates all these mediators in asthma and the exact role of many of them remains uncertain. However, it has been clearly shown that the basic proteins, such as MBP, can cause damage to the bronchial epithelium and that leukotrienes and PAF are potent bronchoconstrictors as well as causing mucus hypersecretion. In addition, eosinophils can generate superoxide radicals as part of the

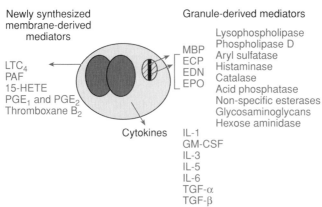

Figure 4.5: Schematic representation of eosinophil-derived mediators, including granule-derived, newly synthesized lipids and cytokines.

oxygen burst. The potential role of these mediators is discussed in more detail in Chapter 5.

Asthmatic airways, particularly in more severe or fatal cases, are characterized by the explosive release of eosinophil granules. The mechanism by which this occurs is not clear. Eosinophils express Fc receptors for IgG, IgA and possibly IgE. Cross-linking of these immunoglobulin receptors is effective in triggering eosinophil degranulation, especially if eosinophils have been primed by mediators such as PAF or IL-5, which on their own are weak secretagogues. Eosinophils are not good at ingesting foreign material and, consistent with their role in protection against parasites, appear to release their mediators more willingly when in contact with a large surface. This secretory process has been described as 'frustrated phagocytosis'. Thus immunoglobulin- or complement-coated beads are particularly effective triggers. In addition, eosinophils only kill parasitic larvae, such as those of *Schistosoma mansoni*, if they have been precoated with either specific immunoglobulin (either IgG, IgA or IgE) or complement (a process called opsonization). However, at present there is little evidence for immunoglobulin- or complement-mediated eosinophil activation in asthmatic airways. The triggers of eosinophil mediator release in asthma are therefore uncertain at present. The known triggers of eosinophil secretion are listed in *Table 4.4*.

4.2.3 The mast cell

Mast cells are tissue-dwelling cells that are widely distributed throughout the body, particularly in the skin, at mucosal surfaces and adjacent to blood vessels. They are characterized by a cytoplasm filled with large granules which stain metachromatically with certain dyes such as toluidine blue. Their granule-filled appearance led Ehrlich, who first described them, to call them *mastzellen* or well-fed cells (*Figure 4.6*). The characteristic staining appearance of mast cells is due to the granules

Table 4.4: Triggers of eosinophil secretion

Fc receptor mediated
IgG-coated particles (Sepharose beads, schistosomula opsonized with specific
   immunoglobulin)
IgA- and surface IgA-coated particles
IgE-coated particles

Complement mediated
C3b through CR1
C3bi through CR3
Opsonized zymosan

Soluble stimuli
For example, PAF, IL-5, RANTES (effective at priming but weak triggers)

being filled with positively charged proteoglycan molecules, either heparin
or chondroitin sulfate.

The high-affinity IgE receptor (FcεRI). Another characteristic feature of
the mast cell, which it shares with the basophil as well as dendritic cells in
the skin (Langerhans cells), is the expression of a high-affinity Fc receptor
for IgE, FcεRI. This is to distinguish it from the low-affinity IgE receptor
FcεRII (CD23), which is more widely expressed and does not bind
monomeric IgE. The affinity of FcεRI for monomeric IgE has a binding
constant of the order of 10^{-10}M compared with 10^{-7}M for most Fc
receptors. The receptor is composed of four chains: an α-chain, which is a
member of the immunoglobulin superfamily and related to IgG Fc

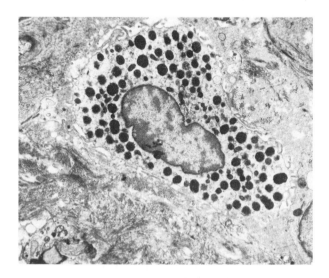

Figure 4.6: Transmission electron micrograph of a mast cell from the human
airway, showing the typical appearance of the cytoplasm full of electron-dense
granules. × 4500. Courtesy of Dr Ann Dewar, National Heart and Lung Institute,
London.

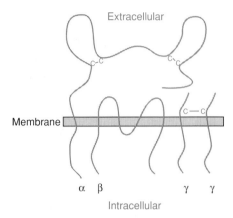

Figure 4.7: Structure of the high-affinity receptor for IgE on mast cells and basophils. It is composed of four chains, α-, β- and two γ-chains. After Metzger (1992).

receptors; a β-chain; and two disulfide-linked γ-chains (*Figure 4.7*). The α-chain binds the Fc region of IgE and the γ-chains are involved in signal transduction. Because of this receptor, mast cells always have IgE bound to their surface even in non-atopic individuals. In atopic individuals some of the surface-bound IgE will recognize allergens to which the individual has been sensitized.

Cross-linking of the IgE receptor, for example by multivalent allergen, results in the release of mast cell-derived mediators, of which histamine is one of the most prominent. This occurs rapidly and is complete within 15 min (*Figure 4.8*). The classic demonstration of this is the wheal and flare reaction seen in skin prick testing of atopic individuals. In this test a drop of allergen, such as grass pollen, is placed on the forearm and the skin lightly scratched with a needle. This exposes the skin mast cells to the allergen. If the subject is atopic and has made IgE directed against the allergen tested then the IgE bound to the mast cells will be cross-linked and the mast cell will degranulate, causing the release of mediators which cause increased vascular permeability and vasodilation: the wheal and flare response. This is both a simple and sensitive test for the presence of specific IgE. In some highly sensitive individuals, if the allergen is injected under the skin there is a risk of large-scale mast cell mediator release leading to anaphylaxis. This is most clearly seen in individuals sensitized to bee or wasp venom, who can develop anaphylactic shock after being stung. If the skin test reaction is sufficiently vigorous (which depends on the dose of allergen, the sensitivity of the individual and how far into the skin the injection is given), inflammatory cells, mononuclear cells, neutrophils and eosinophils are recruited into the skin and a late response occurs.

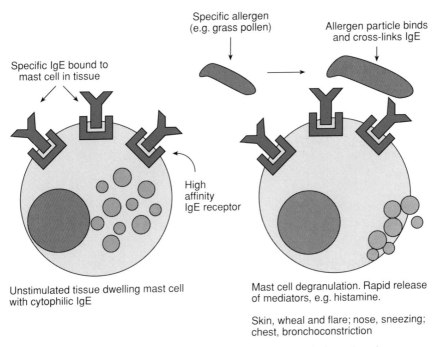

Specific allergen
(e.g. grass pollen)

Allergen particle binds
and cross-links IgE

Specific IgE bound to
mast cell in tissue

High
affinity
IgE receptor

Unstimulated tissue dwelling mast cell
with cytophilic IgE

Mast cell degranulation. Rapid release
of mediators, e.g. histamine.

Skin, wheal and flare; nose, sneezing;
chest, bronchoconstriction

Figure 4.8: Schematic representation of mast cell degranulation. Atopic individuals generate increased amounts of IgE which is bound to the surface of tissue-dwelling mast cells. Contact of the mast cell with the allergen, either by inhalation or through the skin or gut, leads to cross-linking of the IgE, which in turn leads to mast cell degranulation and mediator release. This occurs over 15–30 min and leads to a type 1 hypersensitivity reaction characterized by wheal and flare in the skin, angio-edema in the larynx, sneezing and nasal blockage in the nose, and bronchoconstriction in the lungs.

Mast cell mediators. Like the eosinophil the mast cell can generate a large number of pro-inflammatory mediators on appropriate stimulation. Again like the eosinophil, these include granule-derived and membrane lipid-derived cytokines both preformed and newly formed as a result of protein synthesis (*Table 4.5*). The main granule-derived mast cell mediator is histamine, which is only present in mast cells and basophils. Each mast cell contains picogram quantities of histamine. The effectiveness of anti-histamine drugs (which block the interaction between histamine and one of its receptors, H_1) in treating disease can therefore be used, to some extent, as a marker of the importance of mast cells in that disease. The profile of lipid mediators is similar though not identical to eosinophils. The mast cell is a major potential source of cytokines including TNF-α, IL-4 and IL-5, which, as discussed above, are directly relevant to asthma.

Mast cell heterogeneity. There are two main subgroups of mast cells with important functional differences. These can be most readily distinguished

Table 4.5: Major mast cell-derived mediators

Granule derived
Histamine
Tryptase/chymase
Heparin/chondroitin sulfate

Membrane-derived lipids
LTC_4
5-HETE
LTB_4
PGD_2

Cytokines
IL-4
IL-5
TNF-α

by their content of neutral protease. Mast cells located at mucosal surfaces contain predominantly tryptase, MC_T, whereas mast cells in the deeper connective tissue also contain chymase and carboxypeptidase A, MC_{TC}. Although the functional significance of the different enzyme compositions of the two subtypes is unknown, they can nevertheless be used as markers for the two types of mast cell. There are several other differences between these two cell types (*Table 4.6*). It seems likely that the differences between the mast cell types are determined by the microenvironment in which the cell resides. This was elegantly shown in experiments in which mast cell precursors were implanted into a strain of mouse that is deficient in mast cells (W/W^v mice). When implanted into the stomach the precursors became mucosal-like and in the skin connective tissue-like. It is likely that the differentiation pathway is determined by the cytokines to which the cell is exposed. For example, in humans IL-10 appears to be important in the differentiation of mucosal mast cells.

Table 4.6: Mast cell heterogeneity

Properties	Mucosal mast cell	Connective tissue mast cell
Morphology	Fewer granules of variable size	Many uniform size granules
Protease	Tryptase	Tryptase and chymotryptase
Proteoglycan	Chondroitin sulfate E and heparin	Heparin
Histamine	1.3 pg per cell	15 pg per cell
Response to 48/80	Resistant	Susceptible
Staining	Alcian blue +ve	Safranine +ve
Inhibited by disodium cromoglycate	Yes (BAL mast cell)	No (skin mast cells)

Mast cells and asthma. Mast cells are present through the full thickness of the airways wall, including the epithelium. They are virtually all mucosal

(MC$_T$) type. There is no difference in the number of mast cells in biopsies of the bronchial wall between asthmatic and non-asthmatic controls, although there is a suggestion that in asthmatics the mast cells appear more degranulated. In bronchoalveolar lavage (BAL) samples mast cells are very scanty, making up about 0.02% of the cell population in normals and 0.2% in asthmatics. However, unlike the increase in eosinophils, this is non-specific, being seen in many lung diseases. Indeed, the highest counts are seen in patients with fibrotic lung diseases. There is a suggestion that BAL mast cells in asthma are primed for increased histamine release, although again this may be non-specific.

It has been considered for many years that mast cells are central to the pathogenesis of asthma. Stated simply this hypothesis suggests that inhaled allergen causes mast cell degranulation, which causes immediate, though transient, bronchoconstriction through the release of broncho-constricting mediators such as histamine, leukotriene C$_4$ and PGD$_2$ and more prolonged bronchoconstriction, which mimics clinical asthma, as a result of the recruitment of leukocytes, particularly eosinophils, through the release of specific eosinophil chemoattractants (*Figure 4.9*). The model of these events was the response to allergen inhalation, with the early response corresponding to the initial release of vasoactive and broncho-constricting mediators and the late response corresponding to the inflammatory phase. An important pillar of this hypothesis was the observation in the guinea pig and then in humans that mast cells appeared to release *in vitro* chemotactic factors which were specific for eosinophils. This was called the eosinophil chemotactic factor of anaphylaxis (ECF-a),

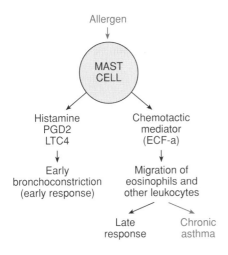

Figure 4.9: Outline of the mast cell hypothesis. Cross-linking of specific IgE on mast cells by inhaled allergen results in mediator release, causing bronchoconstriction and an eosinophil-rich inflammatory response due to the release of eosinophil chemotactic factor of anaphylaxis (ECF-a) and other chemotactic mediators.

and in humans was thought to consist of two tetrapeptides, Val-Gly-Ser-Glu and Ala-Gly-Ser-Glu. However, subsequent work has shown that the ECF-a tetrapeptides have very little activity against eosinophils and that ECF-a in the guinea pig is primarily leukotriene B_4 (LTB_4), a non-selective chemoattractant. There is good evidence that the early events following allergen challenge in the skin, nose or lung are mediated in large part by mast cell-derived mediators. Thus the mast cell-derived mediators histamine, LTE_4 (the terminal metabolite of LTC_4), PGD_2 and tryptase have been detected in increased amounts in BAL fluid a few minutes after allergen challenge. Histamine receptor 1 blockers inhibit the early response by up to 50%, as do receptor antagonists for PGD_2, thromboxane A_2 and leukotriene antagonists. Drugs that inhibit mast cell degranulation such as β_2-agonists and disodium cromoglycate inhibit the early response, whereas corticosteroids, which do not inhibit degranulation, do not. The role of the mast cell in the late response, which is thought to mimic real asthma more closely, is still uncertain. Corticosteroids effectively inhibit this reaction as well as the eosinophil (but not neutrophil) infiltration that accompanies it, whereas β_2-agonists do not. Cromoglycate inhibits, but this drug has multiple anti-inflammatory activities in addition to its effect on mast cells. In clinical asthma there is little conclusive evidence to support a role for mast cells. In particular, histamine receptor 1 blockers are ineffective in treating asthma, unlike seasonal allergic rhinitis (hay fever), in which mast cells clearly have an important role. Disodium cromoglycate is also a relatively ineffective drug in chronic asthma. The weaknesses of the mast cell hypothesis are summarized in *Table 4.7*.

Table 4.7: Problems with the mast cell hypothesis

Does not explain intrinsic asthma
Inhibitors of mast cell degranulation are not very effective in asthma, e.g. Intal-like drugs
Corticosteroids do not block mast cells
No specific increase in mast cells in asthmatic airways
Anti-histamines ineffective in asthma
β_2-Agonists block mast cell degranulation but are not anti-inflammatory

At present the role of the mast cell in asthma is uncertain, although the recent realization that it can generate an array of cytokines including IL-5 and IL-4 is once again moving it center stage. Present evidence would suggest that it is important in initiating the asthmatic process in asthmatics who have a clear allergic component to their asthma. In these circumstances it may also be important in acute severe asthma of sudden onset in brittle asthmatics. There is also evidence for the release of mast cell-derived mediators in exercise-induced asthma and both disodium cromoglycate and β_2-agonists are effective in controlling this variant of the disease.

4.3 Subsidiary cells

4.3.1 Neutrophils

Neutrophils are leukocytes that circulate in the peripheral blood. They are end-stage myelocytes derived from the bone marrow which are recruited into tissue as part of the acute inflammatory response to a wide range of insults. They have a limited capacity for protein synthesis and once in the tissue either die, as part of their cytotoxic role, or become apoptotic and are phagocytosed by macrophages. They are an integral part of the host defense against bacterial infection, as can be seen in the vulnerability to severe infections of patients deficient in neutrophil function as a result of either bone marrow suppression (e.g. in the treatment of leukemia) or an inherited defect such as LAD. Their cytotoxic potential is realized through various lysosomal enzymes, the production of superoxide radicals and an avid capacity for phagocytosis. They can also generate lipid mediators and possess an array of membrane receptors.

Neutrophils are found in normal airways in both biopsies and BAL fluid. Most studies have not found an increase in neutrophils in the airways of chronic asthmatics although they do influx into tissue during the late-phase response. Corticosteroids, which are so effective in asthma, have little effect on neutrophil numbers in either the blood or lungs of asthmatics. There is therefore limited evidence that neutrophils are important in asthma, although they may play a supporting role in the inflammatory response.

4.3.2 Monocytes/macrophages

Monocytes are bone marrow-derived leukocytes that migrate into tissues where they differentiate into larger cells with a similar though distinct phenotype called macrophages which, unlike monocytes, do not stain with peroxidase. They are highly effective phagocytes as well as having the capacity to present antigen to lymphocyte, although in the lung it appears that they may actually suppress antigen presentation by dendritic cells. This could be important in preventing an overreaction to the large amounts of antigen that we inhale. In their phagocytic capacity they have a protective effect against inhaled pathogens and particulate matter as well as removing cellular debris and apoptotic cells. In BAL fluid the majority of cells are macrophages, however most of these are from the alveoli and may therefore have little relevance to asthma. There are resident monocytes/macrophages in the bronchial mucosa which are variably increased in asthma. To an even greater extent than other leukocytes, these cells can generate large amounts of a plethora of inflammatory mediators. Cytokine release by monocytes is effectively inhibited by corticosteroids. Monocytes express a functional Fc receptor for IgE which may be CD23; they can therefore participate directly in allergen-mediated reactions in the airways. Allergen challenge has been shown to result in the release of macrophage-derived mediators in asthmatics, making these cells potential candidates for a pro-inflammatory role in asthma. Despite this, as yet, there is no strong evidence to suggest that this cell is central to the asthmatic response.

4.3.3 Fibroblasts

Fibroblasts are resident in the airways lying just beneath the basement membrane. Airways fibroblasts are specialized in that they contain contractile elements and are therefore called myofibroblasts. Their principal role is to secrete matrix proteins such as collagen and fibronectin, which form the structure of the extracellular tissue. This is continually being remodeled in health and disease so that there is a continuous turnover of these proteins. In certain lung diseases (usually affecting the alveolar compartment of the lung rather than the airways) such as fibrosing alveolitis, there is considerable lung fibrosis with thickening of the lining of the alveolar wall leading to stiff lungs. This is thought to be due to stimulation of fibroblasts by the inflammatory process, resulting in increased production of matrix proteins by these cells. Lung fibrosis is usually associated with irreversible changes. Fibrotic reactions are not a particularly marked feature of the pathology of asthma, although thickening of the collagen layer beneath the epithelial basement membrane is a universal if non-specific finding. This thickening appears to be reversible and its significance to the disease process is uncertain. There is a subgroup of older, non-smoking patients with a history of asthma but relatively fixed airflow obstruction, and it has been suggested that in these patients long-standing inflammation has led to fibrosis of the airways and irreversible obstruction. However, there is little direct evidence for this proposition. Apart from their role in modeling the tissue architecture, fibroblasts like the other cells can produce an array of potentially proinflammatory mediators, particularly cytokine growth factors such as GM-CSF and platelet-derived growth factor as well as the chemotactic peptide IL-8. The extent to which these mediators are generated by fibroblasts in asthmatic airways is as yet unclear.

4.3.4 Epithelial cells

Epithelial desquamation is one of the hallmarks of asthma and is thought to contribute to bronchial hyperresponsiveness through loss of a protective effect, exposing the underlying nerves and subepithelial structures to increased concentrations of inhaled antigens and non-specific irritants. Some studies have demonstrated a good inverse correlation between the epithelial damage and the degree of bronchial hyperresponsiveness, although such studies are open to question because it is difficult to allow for damage due to the biopsy procedure. However, the epithelium is not necessarily a passive cell – it could itself contribute to the inflammation of asthma. Like the cell types described above, epithelial cells can generate a variety of inflammatory mediators, in particular cyclo-oxygenase- and lipoxygenase-derived mediators and various cytokines, including IL-8 and GM-CSF, which could act as chemoattractants or bronchoconstricting agents. In addition, it has been demonstrated that stripping the epithelium from the airways *in vitro* renders the underlying muscle hyperresponsive to bronchoconstricting mediators. This may be due to loss of an epithelial-derived relaxant factor released by epithelial cells, possibly PGE_2. In addition, bronchial epithelium in inflamed airways expresses HLA class II antigens, suggesting it could act as an antigen-presenting cell, especially as under these circumstances it also expresses ICAM-1, the counter-receptor for LFA-1 and an accessory receptor for T-cell activation. However, there does seem an inherent contradiction between a view of the epithelium as a target of eosinophil-mediated damage leading to detachment and death, and a hypothesis that sees the cells of the epithelium as important pro-inflammatory cells directing their own self-destruction. At present the epithelium as victim seems to give a closer fit to the current evidence.

4.3.5 Platelets

Platelets are small cell fragments derived from the disintegration in the bone marrow of megakaryocytes. They circulate in large numbers in the peripheral blood as disk-shaped objects about one-fifth the diameter of a red blood cell. They express a large number of membrane receptors, particularly adhesion receptors, and contain three types of granules, α-granules, dense granules, and lysosomes. The principal function of the platelet appears to be repair of damage to blood vessels and hemostasis. Normally, they circulate singly in the blood vessel but on contact with damaged endothelium they aggregate in large numbers to form the basis of a clot. Abnormalities of platelet function usually lead to bleeding disorders. When stimulated, they generate a large number of mediators some of which, such as PAF, thromboxanes and RANTES, have been implicated in asthma. They are also occasionally seen in the airway mucosa in asthma. This has led some investigators to speculate that they may play a role in the inflammatory process in asthma. However the evidence to support this hypothesis is not at the moment very compelling.

4.4 Conclusion

As in other chronic inflammatory conditions, asthma involves interactions between leukocytes recruited from the peripheral circulation, cells usually resident in tissue, and permanent structures such as in the airways, smooth muscle, nerves, blood vessels and bronchial epithelium. Any inflammatory process is a balance between pro-inflammatory forces and events leading to repair and resolution. It is very much more difficult to study events leading to resolution, so the pro-inflammatory arm tends to be emphasized. In addition, the initiating events in an inflammatory state are often different from the events that lead to its persistence. For example, the response to allergen challenge, which to some degree mimics an attack of asthma, is likely to be mast cell mediated, but this usually resolves rather than progresses to chronic asthma. It could be argued that chronic asthma is therefore due to persistence of allergen exposure. However, it is well recognized that in some occupational asthmatics in whom the triggering agent has been unequivocally identified asthma can persist for many years after total withdrawal from the offending material. Another problem in trying to dissect out the various contributions that each cell type makes to the inflammatory process is that most cell types can release a large variety of mediators, when sufficiently stimulated, which themselves can have a variety of actions. Often commentators are reduced to drawing a complex series of interactions and mediator networks within the airways that throw a doubtful amount of light on the problem.

However, the inflammatory reaction in asthma does have some characteristic features, the most striking of which is the presence of

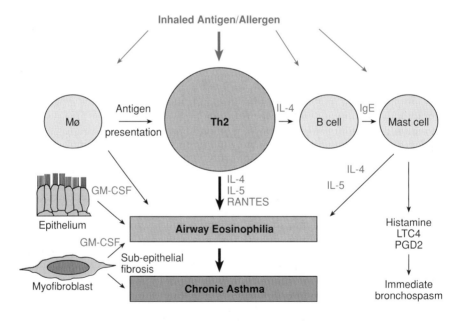

Figure 4.10: Summary of the cellular interactions currently thought to be important in asthma. The major axis is a specific T-cell response to antigen leading to cytokine-induced airway eosinophilia. In atopic asthmatics the Th2 type of lymphocyte subset appears to be responsible, but another type of subset, as yet undefined, generating IL-5 but not IL-4, may be involved in intrinsic asthma. In atopic 'extrinsic' asthma, the inflammatory response is supported by an IgE-mediated mast cell response. Fibroblasts, epithelial cells and macrophage/monocytes could play an accessory role in amplifying the inflammatory response.

eosinophils. The circumstantial evidence that eosinophil-derived mediators cause asthma is strong, although formal proof awaits our ability to
banish them selectively from the airways. In parasitic disease an
eosinophilia is T-cell dependent, and new insights into the ability of T-
cell subsets to secrete differential patterns of cytokines has placed this cell
in the center of events in the asthmatic process. It is also hard to deny the
mast cell some role, at least in the initiation of asthma in atopic
individuals. Taking this into account, a hypothesis to explain the cellular
basis of the inflammatory reaction in asthma, which is supported by
current evidence, is outlined in *Figure 4.10*.

Further reading

General reading

Arm, J.P. and Lee, T.H. (1992) Pathobiology of bronchial asthma. *Adv. Immunol.,*
51, 323–382.

Dale, M.M. and Foreman, J.C. (Eds) (1993) *Textbook of Immunopharmacology*,
3rd Edn. Blackwell Scientific Publications, Oxford.

Kay, A.B. (1991) Asthma and inflammation. *J. Allergy Clin. Immunol.*, **87**, 895–910.

Lymphocytes

Corrigan, C. and Kay, A.B. (1990) CD4 + ve T lymphocyte activation in acute
severe asthma: relationship to disease severity and atopic status. *Am. Rev. Respir.
Dis.*, **141**, 970–977.

Corrigan, C.J. and Kay, A.B. (1992) T cells and eosinophils in the pathogenesis of
asthma. *Immunol. Today*, **13**, 501.

Del Prete, G.F., De Carli, M., Mastromauro, C., Biagiotti, R., Macchia, D.,
Falgiani, P., Ricci, M. and Romagnani, S. (1991) Purified protein derivative of
Mycobacterium tuberculosis and excretory–secretory antigen(s) of *Toxocara canis*
expand *in vitro* human T cells with stable and opposite (type 1 T helper or type 2 T
helper) profile of cytokine production. *J. Clin. Invest.*, **88**, 346–350.

Frew, A.J. and O'Hehir, R. (1992) What can we learn from studies of
lymphocytes present in allergic reaction sites? *J. Allergy Clin. Immunol.*, **89**,
783-788.

Mossman, R. and Coffman, R.L. (1989) Th1 and Th2 cells: different patterns of
lymphokine secretion lead to different functional properties. *Annu. Rev. Immunol.*,
7, 145.

Ricci, M., Ross, O., Bertoni M. and Matucci, A. (1993) The importance of Th2-
like cells in the pathogenesis of airway allergic inflammation. *Clin. Exp. Allergy*,
23, 360–369.

Romagnani, S. (1991) Human Th1 and Th2: doubt no more. *Immunol. Today*, **12**,
256.

Wierenga, E.A., Snoek, M., Jansen, H.M., Bos, J.D., Van Lier, R.A. and Kapsenberg, M.L. (1990) Evidence for compartmentalization of functional subsets of CD4+ve T lymphocytes in atopic patients. *J. Immunol.*, **144**, 4651.

Wierenga, E.A., Snoek, M., De Groot, C., Chretien, I., Bos, J.D., Jansen, H.M. and Kapsenberg, M.L. (1991) Human atopy-specific types 1 and 2 T helper cell clones. *J. Immunol.*, **147**, 2942.

Eosinophils

Gleich, G.J. (1990) The eosinophil and bronchial asthma: current understanding. *J. Allergy. Clin. Immunol.*, **85**, 422.

Gleich, G.J. and Adolphson, C.R. (1986) The eosinophil leukocyte. *Annu. Rev. Immunol.*, **39**, 177.

Makino, S. and Fukuda, T. (Eds) (1992) *Eosinophils. Biological and Clinical Aspects.* CRC Press, Boca Raton.

Smith, H. and Cook, R.M (Eds) (1993) *Immunopharmacology of Eosinophils.* Academic Press, New York.

Spry, C. (1988) *Eosinophils. A Comprehensive Review and Guide to the Scientific and Medical Literature.* Oxford University Press, Oxford.

Wardlaw, A.J. and Kay, A.B. (1987) The role of the eosinophil in the pathogenesis of asthma. *Allergy*, **42**, 321–335.

Weller, P.F. (1991) Immunobiology of eosinophils. *New Engl. J. Med.*, **324**, 1110.

Mast cells

Church, M.K. and Caulfield, J.P. (1992) Mast cell and basophil functions. in *Allergy* (S.T. Holgate and M.K. Church, Eds). Gower Medical Publishing, London, pp. 15.1–15.2.

Foreman, J. (Ed.) (1993) *Immunopharmacology of Mast Cells.* Academic Press, New York.

Holgate, S.T. and Church, M.K. (1992) The mast cell. *Br. Med. Bull.*, **48**, 40–50.

Irani, A.A., Schechter, N.M., Craig, S.S., DeBlois, G. and Schwartz, L.B. (1986) Two types of human mast cells that have distinct neutral protease compositions. *J. Immunol.*, **137**, 962.

Metzzer, H. (1992) The receptor with high affinity for IgE. *Immunol. Rev.*, **125**, 37–48.

Wenzel, S.E., Fowler, A.A. and Schwartz, L.B. (1988) Activation of pulmonary mast cells by bronchoalveolar allergen challenge. *In vivo* release of histamine and tryptase in atopic subjects with and without asthma. *Am. Rev. Respir. Dis.*, **137**, 1002–1008.

Macrophages/monocytes

Adams, D.O. and Hamilton, T.A. (1984) The cell biology of macrophage activation. *Annu. Rev. Immunol.*, **2**, 283.

Aubas, P., Cosso, P., Godard, P., Michel, F.B. and Clot, J. (1984) Depressed suppressor cell activity of alveolar macrophages in bronchial asthma. *Am. Rev. Respir. Dis.*, **130**, 875–878.

Gant, V., Cluzel, M., Shakoor, Z., Rees, P.J., Lee, T.H. and Hamblin, A. (1992) Alveolar macrophage accessory cell function in bronchial asthma. *Am. Rev. Respir. Dis.*, **146**, 900–904.

Lee, T.H. and Lane, S.J. (1992) The role of macrophages in the mechanisms of airway inflammation in asthma. *Am. Rev. Respir. Dis.*, **145**, S27–S30.

Other cells

Allegra, L., Fabbri, L.M., Picotti, G. and Mattoli, S. (1989) Bronchial epithelium and asthma. *Eur. Respir. J.*, **2** (Suppl. 6), 460s–468s.

Barnes, P.J. (1986) Asthma is an axon reflex. *Lancet*, **1**, 242–245.

Hogg, J.C. and Eggleston, P.A. (1984) Is asthma an epithelial disease? *Am. Rev. Respir. Dis.*, **129**, 207–208.

Losewicz, S., Wells, C., Gomez, E., Ferguson, H., Richman, P., Devalia, J. and Davies, R.J. (1990) Morphological integrity of the bronchial epithelium in mild asthmatics. *Thorax*, **45**, 12–15.

Page, C.P. (1988) The involvement of platelets in non-thrombotic processes. *Trends Pharmacol Sci.*, **9**, 66–71.

Roche, W.R. (1991) Fibroblasts and asthma. *Clin. Exp. Allergy*, **21**, 545–548.

Chapter 5

Inflammation in asthma III. The mediators

5.1 Introduction

The pathological and clinical features of inflammation are caused in large part by soluble chemicals either generated from plasma proteins or secreted by cells involved in the inflammatory response. These chemicals bind to membrane receptors, which then transmit a signal into the cell via the pathways discussed in Chapter 3. A considerable array of chemical mediators have been implicated in the inflammatory response. These can be divided into plasma-derived mediators, such as complement, cell-derived mediators, and those derived from the nervous system (neuropeptides). Cell-derived mediators can be further classified into preformed mediators stored in intracellular granules, lipid mediators newly formed from cell membrane phospholipids on cell stimulation, and protein mediators such as cytokines that are newly generated by the cell on activation (*Table 5.1*). Neuropeptides were first described as coming

Table 5.1: Inflammatory mediators

Source	Type	Example
Plasma	Complement	Anaphylotoxins (C5a, C3a)
	Kinins	Bradykinin
Cells	Preformed, granule	Histamine
		Eosinophil basic proteins
	Lipid derived	Leukotrienes
		Platelet-activating factor (PAF)
	Cytokines	IL-5
		IL-4
		RANTES
	Oxygen radicals	Superoxide
		Hydrogen peroxide
Nerves	Neuropeptides	Substance P

from the non-adrenergic, non-cholinergic nervous system and include substance P and vasoactive intestinal peptide.

On the basis of mainly *in vitro* studies, many inflammatory mediators have been implicated in causing asthma. The plethora of potential mediators is further complicated by the fact that any one mediator can have several different functions and can often be generated by many different cell types. There are certain criteria that need to be fulfilled before a mediator can be regarded as likely to play a major role in disease (*Table 5.2*). Relatively few mediators have been demonstrated to meet these criteria to any significant degree. One aim of determining the important mediators in asthma is the hope that specific antagonists will be successful in treating the disease, as is the case with anti-histamines for allergic rhinitis. Whether this is going to be possible or whether asthma is caused by the combined effects of many different mediators remains to be seen. One important point in discussing mediator function is the use of the terms potency, which refers to a concentration of a mediator that causes a given response, and effectiveness, which is the magnitude of the response. A potent mediator is less interesting if its effect is only weak. The potency of a mediator must be related to its likely concentration at the site of inflammation: this is often difficult to ascertain but can be estimated from the amounts generated *in vitro*. Thus LTC_4 is a considerably more potent bronchoconstrictor than histamine, but mast cells produce considerably more histamine than LTC_4 so that the effective concentrations of the two mediators at the site of inflammation may be similar. Another note of caution is in the measurement of inflammatory mediators. Inflammatory mediators are often rapidly metabolized, and present in low concentrations, particularly in plasma, so that accurate and reliable results are difficult to obtain, which may explain why many studies are inconsistent. In addition, measurement of mediators in BAL fluid is complicated because there is a major dilution effect with no satisfactory denominator to compare levels between samples. Thus, unless differences in concentrations of mediators in BAL are considerable and clear-cut, the data needs to be treated with caution.

5.2 Granule-derived mediators

5.2.1 Eosinophil basic proteins

Biochemistry. One of the hallmarks of asthma is an airways eosinophilia.

Table 5.2: Criteria to establish the importance of a mediator in asthma

(1) The functions of the mediator should mimic the pathological changes *in vivo* and *in vitro*
(2) Sufficient amount of the mediator should be generated and secreted in the airways
(3) Inhibition of the mediator's effects should lead to an improvement in the disease
(4) Experimental or clinical deficiency (where it exists) should affect the disease process

Eosinophils are characterized by having about 20 large granules in their cytoplasm, which contain four cationic proteins: major basic protein (MBP), found in the granule core, and eosinophil cationic protein (ECP), eosinophil peroxidase (EPO) and eosinophil-derived neurotoxin (EDN) in the crystalline granule matrix. Although not absolutely specific for eosinophils (basophils contain small amounts of MBP and macrophages and the liver contain EDN), eosinophils are nevertheless the major source of these proteins. It was first noted in the 1970s that eosinophils are able to kill certain helminthic parasites such as opsonized schistosomula of *Schistosoma mansoni*. This activity was found to be due to the toxic effect of the granule proteins, particularly MBP, on the parasite. It was subsequently found that the granule proteins are also toxic for mammalian cells, including bronchial epithelial cells. Toxic effects on epithelium have been reported at concentrations as low as $10\,\mu g\ ml^{-1}$, which are likely to be achieved locally in the airways mucosa in asthma. As was described in Chapter 2, epithelial damage is thought to be a fundamental defect in asthma. The observation that MBP was toxic for airway epithelial cells therefore gave great impetus to the hypothesis that eosinophil-derived mediators are responsible for asthma.

The biochemistry of the basic proteins is summarized in *Table 5.3*. The primary amino acid sequence of MBP deduced from its nucleotide sequence revealed that it contains 17 arginine residues, which explains its basic charge. MBP is synthesized and stored with an acidic N-terminal portion, which is cleaved on secretion, this pro-peptide possibly protecting the cell from the toxic effects of MBP. The mechanism of the cytotoxic effect of MBP is not clear, nor is it clear whether its effects are mediated via specific receptors. On epithelial cells MBP appears to inhibit ATPase activity. Other cationic proteins such as polylysine are able to mimic some of the activities of the basic proteins, such as induction of bronchial hyperresponsiveness, suggesting that the charge properties are important to their activity. EPO is a heme-containing protein that shares 68% identity with neutrophil myeloperoxidase and is particularly toxic when combined with a halide ion such as bromide. ECP is also an arginine-rich protein and is homologous to EDN and pancreatic ribonuclease. It has ribonuclease activity, although the biological significance of this is

Table 5.3: Biochemistry of eosinophil granule basic proteins

	MBP	EPO	EDN	ECP
Mol. mass (kDa)	13.8	14.0 light chain 58.0 heavy chain	16.0	15.6
pl	10.9	11.0	8.9	11.0
Ribonuclease activity	No	No	Yes	Yes
Pro-protein	Yes	Yes	No	No
$\mu g/10^6$ cells	5	15	15	15
Toxic to helminths	Yes	Yes	Variable	Yes
Toxic to epithelium	Yes	Yes	NR	Yes

NR, not reported.

uncertain. The secreted form of ECP differs antigenically from the stored form, the two forms being distinguishable using mAbs, with an antibody called EG1 recognizing the stored form and EG2 the secreted form. These antibodies therefore distinguish resting from actively secreting eosinophils. Transcriptional control over the synthesis of the eosinophil granule proteins has not been investigated in any detail. It is also not clear whether the eosinophil can resynthesize its granule proteins after degranulation or whether there are specific pathways of degradation of the granule proteins.

Basic proteins and asthma. Large amounts of the basic proteins, and particularly MBP, are almost invariably present in the airways of asthmatics dying of status asthmaticus even in the absence of many intact eosinophils. In milder asthmatics, using immunohistology, basic proteins can be detected both within eosinophils and secreted in the tissues. Even very mild asthmatics requiring only occasional inhaled β_2-agonists have increased amounts of MBP in BAL fluid compared with non-asthmatic controls. Inhalation of MBP in non-human primates caused bronchoconstriction and increased bronchial hyperresponsiveness, although this was only seen at high concentrations. It is therefore highly plausible on the present evidence that the eosinophil granule proteins are important in producing some of the tissue abnormalities in asthma.

5.2.2 Histamine

Biochemistry. Histamine was synthesized in 1907 and isolated from ergot in 1910. It is an amine, β-imidazolylethylamine, which is formed from histidine by the action of histadine decarboxylase, an enzyme that is present in the mast cell and basophil. In humans it is stored exclusively in the granules of these cells bound to proteoglycan, either heparin or chondroitin sulfate. It can also be synthesized in large quantities by bacteria such as *Hemophilus influenzae*, which are therefore another source of histamine in biological fluids. Each mast cell contains about 5 pg of histamine. As up to 3% of dispersed lung cells are mast cells, large amounts of histamine could be released into the lung after appropriate stimuli. Histamine can be degraded either by oxidation by diamine oxidase or by methylation to the inactive methylhistamine by histamine methyltransferase (*Figure 5.1*). These enzymes are widely distributed in many tissues. Up to 60% of histamine is released *in vitro* upon degranulation of mast cells or basophils following cross-linking of the IgE receptor.

Histamine has a wide variety of both pro- and anti-inflammatory activities of relevance to asthma (*Table 5.4*). This range of activities is mediated by three histamine receptors whose role has been clarified to a certain extent by specific antagonists, although little is currently known

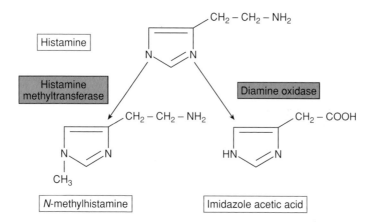

Figure 5.1: Structure of histamine and its metabolites. Histamine is enzymatically metabolized to inactive products by either methylation or oxidation.

about the H_3-receptor. H_1-receptors are primarily responsible for the activities of histamine of relevance to asthma and allergic disease. H_1-antagonists such as Piriton have been available for many years and have played a useful role in the control of allergic symptoms. Their usefulness was limited by causing drowsiness and they have now been largely supplanted by a second generation of more specific, non-sedating potent H_1-antagonists such as terfenadine, astemazole and cetirizine. A major role of H_2-receptors is mediating histamine-induced gastric acid secretion, and H_2-antagonists such as ranitidine and cimetidine have transformed the treatment of peptic ulcers. H_3-receptors are present in the brain, autonomic nervous system, bronchial airways and on mast cells. The distribution of histamine receptors is different between species, which explains in part the considerable differences in the responsiveness of various tissues to histamine between different animals.

Table 5.4: Functions of histamine

Tissue	Effect	Receptor subtype
Bronchial smooth muscle	Bronchoconstriction	H_1
Pulmonary arteries	Constriction	H_1
	Dilatation	H_2
Bronchial arteries	Dilatation	H_1 (low dose)
Bronchial venules	Increased permeability	H_1
Nasal vessels	Dilatation and increased permeability	H_1
Sputum	Increased volume	H_1
	Increased glycoprotein	H_2
Leukocytes	Generally inhibitory actions, e.g. inhibition of basophil histamine release	H_2

Histamine and asthma. Inhaled histamine causes bronchoconstriction by a combination of a direct effect on bronchial smooth muscle and through increased vagal tone. Asthmatics have increased responsiveness to histamine; indeed, this is the basis for the Pc20 measurement of non-specific bronchial hyperresponsiveness. Histamine-induced bronchoconstriction develops over 2–5 min with a duration of action of 20 min. It accounts for up to 50% of the fall in lung function seen during the early response to allergen challenge. Several types of assays are available for the detection of histamine in body fluids (*Table 5.5*). Measurement in plasma is very difficult because of proteins causing high background interference, low concentrations of histamine, which in any case is rapidly metabolized, and the problem of contamination with histamine from basophils. Nevertheless, increased concentrations of histamine have been detected in circumstances associated with mast cell degranulation, such as urticaria, systemic mastocytosis and during the early response following allergen challenge. Studies in clinical asthma have been variable, with some demonstrating evidence of increased concentrations of histamine in plasma or BAL fluid and other studies showing no increase. Considering the difficulties in measuring histamine and the problem of allowing for variable dilution effects when measuring concentrations of mediator levels in BAL fluid, the assembled data are unconvincing as evidence for a major role of histamine in asthma. Even more damning is the lack of therapeutic efficacy of potent anti-histamines. Despite providing some benefit in allergic rhinitis, H_1-receptor blockers are largely ineffective in the treatment of both chronic asthma and acute severe asthma. Because of this it has been concluded that, despite being an important mediator in type I immediate hypersensitivity reactions, current evidence provides little support for an important role for histamine in asthma. This observation, as discussed earlier, has had important consequences for the evaluation of the role of mast cells in the pathogenesis of asthma.

5.3 Lipid mediators

Lipid mediators are not stored in cells but generated *de novo*, when the cell is stimulated, from membrane phospholipids by the action of membrane-

Table 5.5: Histamine assays

Assay	Sensitivity	Uses
Bioassay using guinea pig ileum	Sensitive	Cumbersome. Confirms functional activity of histamine
Automated fluorometric method	Insensitive (6 ng ml^{-1})	Analysis of large numbers of samples
Single-isotope radioimmunoassay	Sensitive (0.5 ng ml^{-1}) and specific	Moderate numbers of samples
Double-isotope radioimmunoassay	Highly sensitive and specific	Laborious, measurement of plasma samples

Table 5.6: Principal cell sources of lipid mediators in man

	$LTC_4/D_4/E_4$	LTB_4	PAF	PGD_2
Mast cells	+ +	+/−	−	+ +
Basophils	+ +	+/−	−	−
Eosinophils	+ +	−	+ +	−
Neutrophils	−	+ +	+ +	−
Monocytes/ macrophages	−	+ +	+ +	−
Platelets	−	−	+ +	−

bound phospholipases. Lipid mediators are produced in variable amounts by a number of cell types (*Table 5.6*). Phospholipids have the common structure of a three-carbon glycerol backbone with fatty acid chains of variable length on carbons-1 and -2 and a phosphate group on carbon-3, to which a base such as choline is attached (*Figure 5.2*). Fatty acids are carbon chains of variable length with a terminal carboxyl (COOH) group, which is either saturated (i.e. has no double bonds) or unsaturated. They are attached to the glycerol backbone by acyl or alkyl linkages. There are two main groups of lipid mediators of potential importance in asthma. The eicosanoids, which are 20-carbon fatty acids derived from arachidonic acid, and platelet-activating factor (PAF). Arachidonic acid is mainly derived directly from the diet, whence it is taken into the cell and attached to phospholipids by an acyltransferase enzyme.

5.3.1 Arachidonic acid-derived mediators (eicosanoids)

Arachidonic acid is a major component of membrane phospholipids, usually phosphatidylcholine, and is cleaved from these lipids by the action

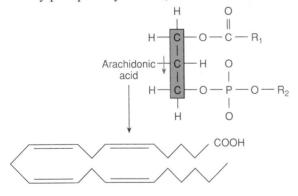

⟶ Site of action of phospholipase A_2

Figure 5.2: Arachidonic acid is cleaved from membrane glycerophospholipids by the action of phospholipase A_2. Glycerophospholipids, found mainly in the cell membrane or in cytoplasmic lipid bodies, have a three-carbon backbone to which fatty acid chains are attached at the carbon-1 and -2 positions and a phosphate group at the carbon-3 position.

of phospholipase A_2, which is activated when a cell becomes triggered. The free arachidonic acid is then metabolized in the membrane into members of the prostaglandin family by the action of the enzyme cyclo-oxgenase and to members of the leukotriene family by the action of the enzyme 5-lipoxygenase. There are a number of related enzymes such as 12- and 15-lipoxygenase that produce mediators related to the leukotrienes called hydroxyeicosatetranoic acids (HETEs) but these are of uncertain physiological significance and relevance to asthma (*Figure 5.3*).

Leukotriene biochemistry. There are two types of leukotrienes, so named because they were initially detected in leukocytes: the sulfidopeptide leukotrienes, formerly called the slow-reacting substance of anaphylaxis (SRS-A), whose principal action is bronchoconstriction; and leukotriene B_4, which is a leukocyte chemoattractant and activator. The biosynthesis and chemical structure of these mediators are shown in *Figure 5.4*. 5-Lipoxygenase is active only in the presence of an 18 kDa membrane protein called 5-lipoxygenase-activating protein (FLAP), which binds to arachidonic acid and makes it available to 5-lipoxygenase. Further oxygenation of arachidonic acid leads to a class of compounds called the lipoxins, but there is little evidence to date that they play a role in asthma. The principal cell sources of the leukotrienes are shown in *Table 5.6*. The three sulfidopeptide leukotrienes are all biochemically active and are

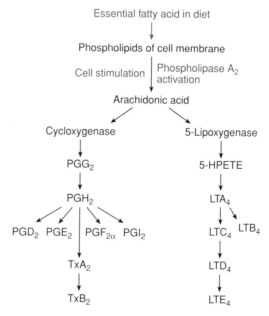

Figure 5.3: Cascade of events leading to the generation of the eicosanoid mediators. Arachidonic acid cleaved from membrane phospholipids gives rise to either prostanoids as a result of the action of the enzyme cyclo-oxygenase or leukotrienes as a result of 5-lipoxygenase activity. The initial products 5-HPETE, LTA_4, PGG_2 and PGH_2 are unstable.

generated in sequence: LTC$_4$, LTD$_4$, then LTE$_4$. LTC$_4$ is rapidly converted to LTD$_4$ and LTE$_4$ by the action of glutamyl transpeptidases and dipeptidases present in cell membranes, secreted cellular granules and plasma. Approximately 40% of LTC$_4$ is converted to LTD$_4$ within 30 min. All three leukotrienes can be readily oxidized to inactive catabolites.

Leukotriene B$_4$ is a potent and effective leukocyte chemoattractant and activating mediator priming granulocytes for enhanced functions,

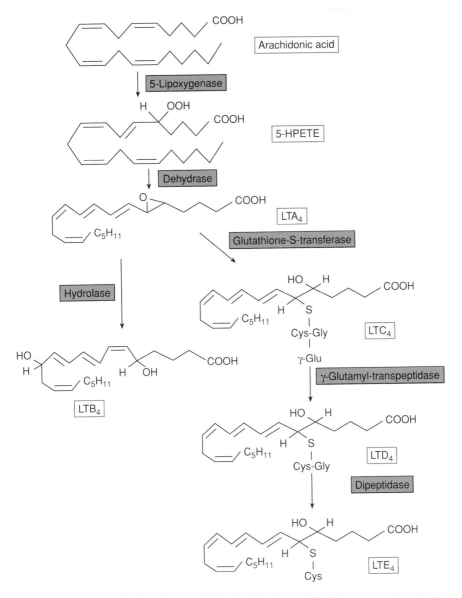

Figure 5.4: Biosynthetic pathway of the leukotrienes with the enzymes involved shown in boxes. FLAP, 5-lipoxygenase-activating protein. Cysteine (Cys), Glycine (Gly), Glutamic acid (Glu).

including cytotoxicity, mediator release and adhesion. It is active on eosinophils and neutrophils *in vitro*, although studies of *in vivo* administration have reported only neutrophil accumulation. Leukotrienes C_4, D_4 and E_4 have a different set of activities, causing bronchial smooth muscle constriction *in vitro* and bronchoconstriction on inhalation in both asthmatics and normal subjects. Bronchoconstriction develops over 30 min and lasts 2 h. As is the case with other bronchoconstricting mediators, asthmatics are more sensitive to the leukotrienes, particularly LTE_4, than normal subjects. The sulfidopeptide leukotrienes can also cause an increased responsiveness to histamine and methacholine, although this response appears to be variable and relatively short-lived compared with the increase seen after allergen challenge or during natural exposure of sensitized individuals to grass pollen during the hay fever season. Other effects of the sulfidopeptide leukotrienes of relevance to asthma include increased mucus production and vascular permeability. In a recent report, inhalation of LTE_4 was found to cause a marked BAL eosinophilia. The significance of this interesting observation is currently uncertain.

Leukotrienes and asthma. Antibodies to some of the leukotrienes are available, and amounts of these mediators can be measured in biological fluids by immunoassay. Some of the antibodies cross-react and measurements ideally need to be supported by chromatography to confirm the exact identity of the leukotriene detected. The rapid metabolism of LTC_4 and LTD_4 to LTE_4 makes this last species the best one to measure. A number of studies have found increased amounts of sulfidopeptide leukotrienes in BAL fluid, plasma and urine. Increased amounts of LTE_4 have been found in the urine after allergen challenge, and during acute severe asthma and steady-state asthma. Studies using leukotriene antagonists have suggested that about 30–50% of the early response to allergen challenge is due to leukotrienes. A number of effective leukotriene antagonists and 5-lipoxygenase inhibitors are now becoming available, which should give more information on the role of the leukotrienes in asthma (see Chapter 7). There is less evidence of a role for leukotriene B_4 in asthma. It is most clearly recognized as a neutrophil-activating mediator and therefore may not play a central role in the disease.

Prostanoid biochemistry. The inflammatory mediators derived from arachidonic acid by the action of cyclo-oxygenase (loosely termed prostanoids) include the prostaglandins, so named because they were first detected in the prostate gland, thromboxanes and prostacyclin. Their biosynthesis is illustrated in *Figure 5.5*. They have a variety of effects and have been detected in a number of inflammatory conditions. Aspirin and related non-steroidal anti-inflammatory drugs (NSAIDs) block cyclo-oxygenase, and their anti-inflammatory, antipyretic and analgesic

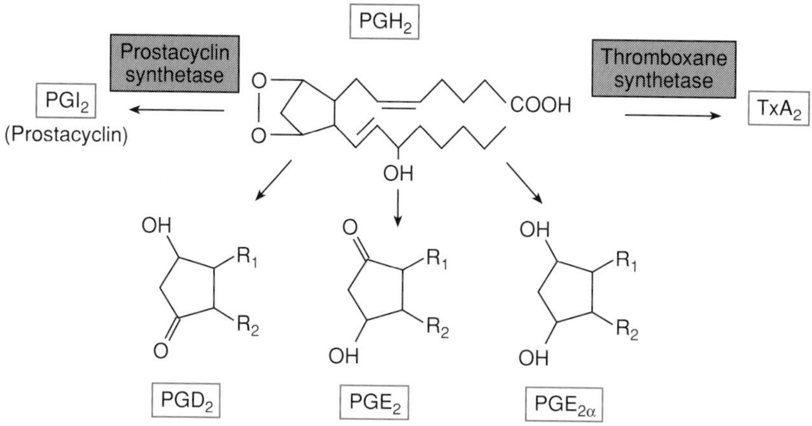

Figure 5.5: Structure of the prostanoids and the enzymes involved in prostacyclin and thromboxane synthesis. PGH_2 is unstable and is rapidly metabolized to PGD_2, PGE_2 and $PGF_{2\alpha}$. The distinct ring structures of these three compounds are shown.

activities are a testament to the functions of these mediators. The fever-inducing actions of IL-1 are thought to be due to the release of PGE_2. Cyclo-oxygenase occurs in most mammalian cells and is located in the endoplasmic reticulum. The nomenclature of the prostanoid family is confusing and derived from their original description. For example, prostaglandin E was so called because it is soluble in ether and prostaglandin F because it is soluble in buffer (*fostat* in Swedish); the suffix attached to these names refers to the number of double bonds. Prostanoids are rapidly metabolized enzymatically with a half-life in the blood of less than 1 min. The lung and kidney are particularly rich in these catabolic enzymes, with 90% of an infusion of prostaglandins metabolized during a single passage through perfused lungs.

Prostanoids and asthma. The main effect of prostanoids relevant to asthma is on airways smooth muscle. PGD_2, $PGF_{2\alpha}$ and thromboxane A_2 (TxA_2) cause bronchoconstriction and a transient increase in bronchial hyperresponsiveness, whereas PGE_2 and PGI_2 cause relaxation of bronchial smooth muscle. PGD_2 is generated in large amounts by mast cells and has been detected in increased amounts in BAL fluid from asthmatics after allergen challenge, as have increased amounts of thromboxane B_2 (TxB_2), the stable metabolite of TxA_2. For most prostanoids there are no specific inhibitors, so a full analysis of their role in asthma is not yet possible. Some studies using a combination of thromboxane synthesis inhibitors and thromboxane A_2 analogs have implicated TxA_2 in the pathogenesis of airways hyperresponsiveness in asthmatics as well as the late response to allergen challenge. However, other studies have found no effect of TxA_2 synthetase inhibitors on either the bronchoconstriction or increased hyperresponsiveness following allergen challenge. Moreover, the lack of any consistent effect of cyclo-oxygenase inhibitors on either airways hyperresponsiveness or airway caliber in clinical asthma makes it unlikely that cyclo-oxygenase mediators are important as pro-inflammatory mediators in the pathogenesis of asthma.

5.3.2 Platelet-activating factor (PAF)

Biochemistry. PAF was first detected in the early 1970s as a factor released from antigen-challenged basophils that was able to aggregate platelets, hence its name. Some 7 years later it was fully characterized and found to be a lipid with the structure 1-*O*-alkyl-2-acetyl-*sn*-glycero-3-phosphocholine with the alkyl carbon chain being usually composed principally of 16 carbon atoms (*Figure 5.6*). It is now known to have a range of functions and to be synthesized by many cell types, although it is not secreted in large amounts by either human basophils or mast cells (*Table 5.7*).

In leukocytes the main pathway of biosynthesis is the acetylation of lyso-PAF generated by cleavage of an acyl group (often arachidonic acid) from the C-2 position of 1-*O*-alkyl-glycerophospholipids. PAF is not stored, but like the eicosanoids is generated *de novo* on cell stimulation.

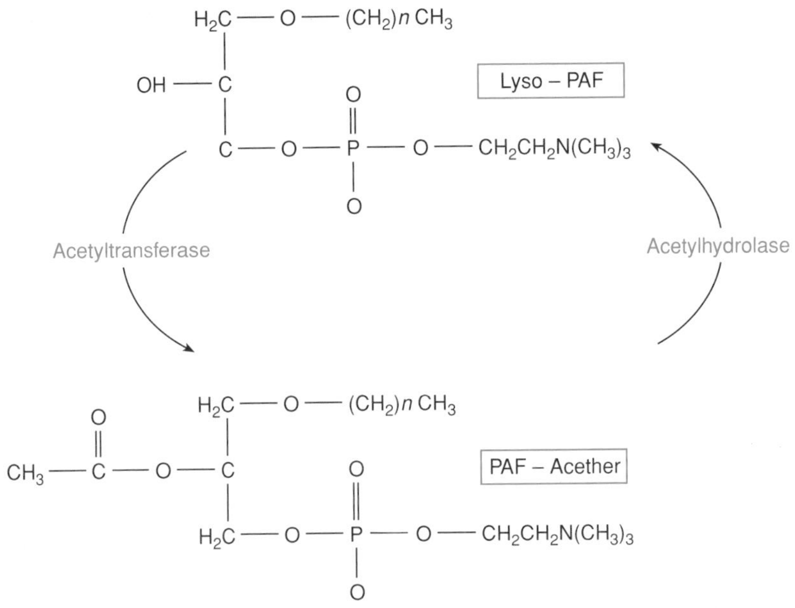

Figure 5.6: Chemical structure of PAF and its inactive precursor lyso-PAF, with the enzymes involved in its biosynthesis and metabolism. PAF is a glycerophospholipid with an alkyl ether group at the carbon-1 position (C-O-CH_2-CH_2), an acetyl group at the C-2 position (C-O-CO-CH_2) and a phosphocholine group at the C-3 position. The carbon chain at C-1 is 16–18 carbons in length.

Table 5.7: Functions of PAF

Airways
Bronchoconstriction
Prolonged increase in BHR in normal subjects (variable)
Increased secretion of mucus
Increased vascular permeability leading to edema
Leukocyte activation
Priming of neutrophils, eosinophils and monocytes
Mediator of secretion in previously primed cells
Chemotaxis of neutrophils, eosinophils and monocytes
Recruitment of neutrophils and eosinophils into skin and lung
Platelet aggregation and secretion

Biodegradation involves hydrolysis back to lyso-PAF by the actions of an acetylhydrolase. Such a hydrolase is present in human plasma and found in the cytoplasm of a number of cells, which means that PAF is rapidly metabolized to an inactive form. PAF is also rapidly metabolized when perfused through the lung. Much of the PAF generated by a cell on stimulation remains cell associated. The relevance of this is unclear, although it could be acting as an intracellular messenger or binding to its own PAF receptor and acting as a self-mediator (autocrine). There is also evidence that endothelial cell-associated PAF can stimulate leukocyte binding to the endothelium. This direct cell-to-cell form of transmission may explain how PAF can exert its effects despite being rapidly metabolized in biological fluids.

PAF was originally measured using the aggregation of rabbit platelets as a biological assay. This was a sensitive but technically demanding assay and has now been superseded by immunoassays. Being a lipid it was thought that PAF might interact with a cell by becoming incorporated into phospholipid. However, at least one specific receptor for PAF has been fully characterized.

PAF and asthma. PAF has a number of biological effects of relevance to asthma. In particular, its ability to cause non-specific bronchial hyperresponsiveness for up to 2 weeks after a single inhalation, and the observations that it is a highly effective eosinophil chemoattractant and priming agent, led to suggestions that it is of major importance in the pathogenesis of asthma. As a result, a number of potent receptor antagonists have been developed and are now in early clinical trials (discussed in Chapter 7). However, enthusiasm for PAF has waned with the realization that the effects of PAF on bronchial hyperresponsiveness are weak, inconsistent and not seen in asthmatics. In addition, it has not been possible to detect increased amounts of PAF in asthma, and the results of the preliminary clinical trials with PAF antagonists have been disappointing. The ability of PAF to act in direct cell-to-cell contacts suggests that an inhibitor of PAF synthesis may be more effective than a receptor antagonist.

5.4 Cytokines

Cytokines are a large group of peptide mediators secreted by many cells with a wide range of biological effects *in vitro*. While T lymphocytes and monocytes are generally regarded as the principal sources for many cytokines, other cells including eosinophils, mast cells, fibroblasts and endothelial cells can produce substantial quantities of some cytokines. They are soluble chemicals that interact with target cells via specific membrane receptors. Their action, unlike say endocrine hormones, is thought to be relatively short range, but it seems likely that what are called cytokine networks form an intricate pattern of signals that control many aspects of cellular function in both health and disease. There is no very good classification system for cytokines because of their hetero-geneity and multitude of effects. In addition, many cytokines were named on the basis of their original cell source or function, which may no longer be the most important or relevant. *Table 5.8* outlines the major groups of cytokines. There is still relatively little evidence of a role for many

Table 5.8: Cytokines

Type	Example	Comment
Hemopoietic growth factors, colony-stimulating factors (CSF)	GM-CSF G-CSF IL-5	Also prime mature leukocytes
Tissue growth factors	Epithelial growth factor (EGF) Platelet-derived growth factor (PGDF) Fibroblast growth factor (FGF)	Actions not restricted to tissue associated with name
Interleukins (IL)	IL-1 IL-2	Defined as lymphocyte growth factors but usually many actions with lymphocyte stimulation often not major action
Chemokines	RANTES IL-4	Family of 6- to 10-kDa chemoattractants with relatively selective activity. Two subfamilies (C-X-C and C-C) based on conserved cysteine residues
Others	Tumor necrosis factors Transforming growth factor beta (TGF-β) family Interferons	Each group has 2–4 closely related members. Diverse functions

cytokines in asthma, although it is possible that fibroblast growth factors are responsible for the thickening of the collagen layer beneath the basement membrane and that TNF-α and IL-1, both generated by mast cells, monocytes and eosinophils, could be important in up-regulating adhesion molecules on endothelial cells. There is more direct evidence for the importance of one group of related cytokines in asthma. These are the cytokines IL-3, IL-4, IL-5 and GM-CSF, which are each located on the long arm of chromosome 6 and secreted together by Th2-type lymphocytes. They have related functions which are summarized in *Table 5.9.*

Table 5.9: Th2 lymphocyte-associated cytokines

Name	Principal cell source (other cell sources)	Mol.mass (kDa)	Functions of relevance to asthma
IL-5	T lymphocytes (mast cells, eosinophils)	40	Selective eosinopoiesis Primes and prolongs survival of mature eosinophils Eosinophil tissue accumulation *in vivo*?
IL-4	T lymphocytes (mast cells, basophils)	15–19	IgE production by B cells Stimulation of Th2 cells Inhibition of Th1 cells Eosinophil tissue accumulation *in vivo* (transgenic mice) Selective up-regulation of VCAM-1 on vascular endothelial cells
GM-CSF	Monocytes, T lymphocytes (eosinophils, epithelial cells and many other cells)	18–22	Primes and prolongs survival of mature eosinophils (non-selective) Non-selective eosinopoiesis
IL-3	T lymphocytes (eosinophils, mast cells)	15–25	Mast cell growth As for GM-CSF

5.4.1 Interleukin 5 (IL-5)

IL-5 is of particular interest because it has such a restricted function, being a growth factor for eosinophils and possibly basophils as well as stimulating the function of mature eosinophils and basophils (in mice it also acts on B cells). It is produced principally by T lymphocytes, although there is some evidence for it being secreted by eosinophils and mast cells. IL-5 is a disulfide-linked, homodimeric glycoprotein with a molecular mass of about 40 kDa and a primary structure comprising 115 amino acids. Dimerization in a head-to-tail configuration is essential for activity. *In vitro* studies suggested that IL-5 is involved only in the terminal differentiation of eosinophils and that other growth factors are required to promote the growth of earlier precursors. However, transgenic mice which were engineered to overproduce IL-5 had a profound eosinophilia without any increase in the production of other eosinophil growth factors. Thus, IL-5 alone appears to be able to cause eosinophil differentiation from early precursors to the mature cell. This would be consistent with the eosinophilia seen, without expansion of the other leukocyte lineages, in asthma and parasitic disease. This is of considerable importance, for it suggests that blocking IL-5 function alone may abolish eosinophil growth, and if eosinophils are indeed a key cell in asthma such a strategy should be an effective treatment. Further support for this approach comes from studies in parasitized mice in which anti-IL-5 mAbs abolish the parasite-induced eosinophilia. Interestingly, transgenic mice with high eosinophil counts in both blood and tissue were perfectly healthy. This emphasizes the fact that increased numbers of circulating eosinophils are insufficient on their own to produce tissue damage: a trigger is also required to cause eosinophil mediator release.

5.4.2 Interleukin 4 (IL-4)

IL-4 is a 129 amino acid polypeptide with a molecular mass in the region of 18 kDa. It was first described as a B-cell growth factor, although the receptor for IL-4 is expressed on a number of other cells, including endothelial cells, T cells and mast cells. It has a number of activities of relevance to asthma, including its role as a major factor responsible for isotype switching of B cells to make IgE. IL-4 stimulates endothelial cells to express VCAM-1 without increasing expression of other endothelial adhesion molecules and promotes transmigration of eosinophils in a VLA-4-dependent fashion. IL-4, when added to antigen-stimulated mononuclear cells, promotes the generation of Th2-type cytokines and inhibits Th1 production. It therefore has reciprocal actions to IFN-γ, which inhibits Th2 cells and stimulates Th1 cytokine production. These actions appear to be relevant *in vivo*, at least in mice. Balb/c mice, when infected with the parasite *Leishmania major*, generate a Th2 pattern of cytokines with high IgE and an eosinophilia. A related strain of mice, C57BL/6, produces IFN-γ and IL-2 with no IgE or eosinophils. Anti-IL-4 mAb or IFN-γ, when administered to the Balb/c mice prior to infection, produces a Th1-type phenotype. IL-4 transgenic mice, which are genetically engineered to produce large amounts of IL-4, have high IgE levels and a tissue eosinophilia. Moreover, unlike the IL-5 transgenic mice they are unwell and have an inflammatory response in the eyes which has similar features to allergic conjunctivitis. Mice in which the IL-4 gene has been genetically disabled (IL-4 knockout mice) are unable to mount an IgE response to infection with *Nippostrongylus brasiliensis*, and also have impaired production of IL-5 and IL-10 (a Th2-cell associated cytokine in mice but not humans) and a markedly reduced eosinophilic response to infection. Lastly, treatment of the nasal mucosa with corticosteroids sufficient to inhibit an allergic response to allergen challenge was associated with loss of expression of IL-4 mRNA in the nasal mucosa, while there was no change in IL-5 mRNA expression. IL-4 is therefore being increasingly seen as central to the allergic response. IL-4 as well as IL-5 is generated in the airways in allergic individuals, and mast cells contain large amounts of IL-4 stored in granules and released on mast cell degranulation. It is not clear whether IL-4 is involved in intrinsic asthma where IgE levels are low.

5.4.3 Chemokines

Another important family of cytokines is the chemokines. These consist of 6 to 10 kDa proteins that are between 20 and 45% similar in amino acid sequence. They are highly effective leukocyte chemoattractants and priming agents. They are basic polypeptides that are strongly bound by heparin and therefore may be difficult to measure in biological fluids where mast cell degranulation has occurred. The cDNA for these cytokines revealed a common four-cysteine motif in the primary structure. The family can be divided into two subsets. One subset, typified by IL-8, is located on chromosome 4 and is generally more active on neutrophils than mononuclear cells. The second subset, typified by a mediator called RANTES, is located on chromosome 17 and is more active on mononuclear cells. In the IL-8 subset the first two conserved cysteines that make up the family motif are separated by an amino acid residue (C-X-C subfamily), whereas in the RANTES subfamily the cysteines are adjacent (C-C; see *Table 5.10*). Of particular interest has been the exciting observation that RANTES is a highly effective chemo-attractant and priming agent for both eosinophils and memory CD4 + ve T lymphocytes, so that it has the appropriate profile of activity to be involved in eosinophil recruitment into the lung. RANTES is secreted by antigen-stimulated T cells and platelets. However, whether it is generated in allergic inflammation is not currently known.

5.5 Mediator receptors

5.5.1 Chemotactic receptors

A number of receptors for chemotactic mediators have been cloned, and

Table 5.10: Chemokines

C-X-C	C-C
IL-8	RANTES
Platelet factor 4 (PF4)	MIP-1α
β-TG	MIP-1β
MGSF	MCP-1

MGSF, melanoma growth-stimulating factor; β-TG, β-thromboglobulin; MCP-1 monocyte chemotactic protein 1.

despite the diverse chemical nature of the mediators the receptors all appear to be members of the G-protein-linked superfamily. These receptors, a prototype member of which was the receptor for rhodopsin, are characterized by having seven putative membrane-spanning domains and conserved cysteine residues in the first and second extracellular loops (*Figure 5.7*). As well as chemoattractants, members of the family include β-adrenoreceptors, the muscarinic acetylcholine receptor, hormone receptors such as the thyrotropin receptor, and neuropeptide receptors such as the substance K and VIP receptors. There is 23–32% amino acid identity between the receptors for IL-8, macrophage inflammatory protein 1α (MIP1α), f-MLP (a bacterial-derived chemotactic peptide) and C5a, with the chemokine receptors being more closely related. The G-protein-linked nature of these receptors is consistent with the observation that functions induced by chemoattractants are inhibited by either pertussis or cholera toxin, which inhibit G-proteins.

5.5.2 Cytokine receptors

Although chemokines are cytokines, their receptors differ from other cytokines. Whereas chemokine receptors are single-chain proteins with several transmembrane regions, most cytokines have a one- or two-polypeptide structure, each with a single transmembrane domain. Cytokine receptors are classified into five subgroups according to structural homology (*Table 5.11*). Type 1 receptors have an extracellular domain of about 210 amino acids. They have a conserved motif containing cysteine and tryptophan residues at their N terminal end and another conserved motif at their C terminal end (W (tryptophan)-S (serine)-X(non-conserved)-W-S).

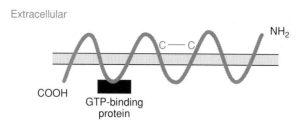

Figure 5.7: Schematic outline of the structure of the chemotactic receptors. They are characterized by seven putative transmembrane regions predicted from their content of hydrophobic amino acids. These regions are thought to form a ligand-binding pocket (not shown in this representation), although conservation of the N-terminal region between chemokine receptors that can bind common chemokines suggests that the N-terminal region is also important in this respect. The G-protein is thought to be associated with the third intracellular loop, and two cysteines in the second and third extracellular loops are highly conserved and considered to form a covalent bond important to the integrity of the receptor.

Table 5.11: Cytokine receptors

Type	Receptors for	Structure
1	Most interleukins	Approximately 210-amino-acid extracellular domain
	GM-CSF	One or two heterodimeric chains
	G-CSF	Growth factor receptors without a tyrosine kinase domain
2	IFN-α/β	Chromosome 6: single-chain (although linked to
	IFN-γ	other as yet uncharacterized chains)
3	TNF-α and -β	Single chain: cysteine-rich extracellular domain
	CD40	
4	IL-1	Immunoglobulin like
5	EGF	Growth factor receptors with a cytoplasmic domain
	PDGF	that encodes tyrosine kinase activity (i.e. leads to phosphorylation of proteins on tyrosine)
		Large extracellular ligand-binding domain

Of particular interest in terms of asthma are the receptors for the Th2-associated cytokines IL-4, IL-5, IL-3 and GM-CSF. These are all type 1 cytokine receptors. The IL-3, IL-5 and GM-CSF receptors are hetero-dimers, with a distinct α chain and a common β chain (*Figure 5.8*). The IL-4 receptor is a single chain 140-kDa polypeptide resulting in a single class of high-affinity receptors (K_d = 20–80 pM). It has a large cytoplasmic domain of 569 amino acids. As well as being expressed on leukocytes, it is expressed on a wide variety of non-hemopoietic cells, including fibro-blasts, neuroblasts and keratinocytes.

5.6 Other mediators

A large number of other inflammatory mediators have been discussed

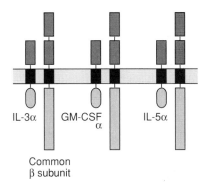

Figure 5.8: Schematic outline of the structure of the related receptors for IL-3, IL-5 and GM-CSF. They each have distinct α-chains which bind the cytokine with low affinity (except the α chain of the IL-5 receptor, which binds with a relatively high affinity), and a common β-chain that does not itself bind any of the cytokines but confers high affinity on each of the receptors. The β-chain is thought to be involved in signal transduction. The common β-chain and the α-chains each have extracellular domains, indicated by the shaded boxes (two in the case of the β-chain), which contain the motifs found in the type 1 cytokine receptor family.

over time in the context of asthma pathogenesis. These include neuropeptides, components of the kinin system, adenosine, components of the complement system, and oxygen radicals.

5.6.1 Neuropeptides

In addition to the sympathetic and cholinergic nervous systems there is an alternative non-adrenergic non-cholinergic (NANC) system, which is mediated by a large number of small peptides called neuropeptides. Neuropeptides appear to be contained within cholinergic or adrenergic nerves rather than forming an alternative neural pathway. Neuropeptides modulate smooth muscle tone, vascular tone and permeability, and mucus gland secretion. Some neuropeptides, such as vasoactive intestinal peptide (VIP), have generally inhibitory effects, whereas others such as substance P cause bronchoconstriction and stimulate mucus gland secretion. Nitric oxide, although not a neuropeptide, appears to mediate some of the NANC-mediated bronchodilator effects. The effects of neuropeptides with particular relevance to asthma are summarized in *Table 5.12*. Epithelial shedding is a hallmark of asthma, and this desquamation exposes the sensory nerves which might then be chronically overstimulated in asthma. This, together with the wide distribution of neuropeptides in the airways and their potent effects on airway physiology, has suggested a role in asthma by either overproduction of excitatory neuropeptides or increased degradation of inhibitory ones. However, although it seems likely that neuropeptides are important in maintaining the homeostasis of the airways milieu, a place for these neurotransmitters in asthma pathogenesis remains highly speculative. It is hoped that the development of specific antagonists will help to clarify the importance of this family of mediators.

5.6.2 Kinins

Kinins are generated from kininogens, which consist of two proteins, high- and low-molecular-weight kininogen, synthesized from a single gene

Table 5.12: Functions of neuropeptides of relevance to asthma

Neuropeptide	Function
Vasoactive intestinal peptide (VIP)	Relaxation of bronchial smooth muscle: mainly large airways
	Stimulation of mucus secretion from submucosal glands
	Vasodilation of bronchial vessels
Tachykinins (substance P, NKA)	Bronchial smooth muscle constriction *in vitro* and *in vivo*
	Stimulation of mucus secretion
	Vasodilation
Calcitonin gene-related peptide (CGRP)	Vasodilation
Gastrin releasing peptide (GRP)	Stimulation of mucus secretion

by alternative splicing. Kininogens are synthesized in the liver and circulate in plasma, where they are metabolized to the physiologically active kinins bradykinin and lysylbradykinin, by the action of either plasma or tissue kallikrein, which are biochemically distinct molecules. Tissue kallikrein is present in the airways, and kinins have been detected in increased amounts in subjects with asthma and rhinitis after allergen challenge to both upper and lower airways. Bradykinin and lysylbradykinin are interesting in that they cause bronchoconstriction in asthmatics but not normal controls. This appears to be an indirect effect, possibly mediated via neural reflexes, as bradykinin is only a weak bronchoconstrictor of isolated airway muscle. Again, direct evidence for a role for kinins in asthma awaits the development of potent antagonists.

5.6.3 Adenosine

Another mediator that causes bronchoconstriction in asthmatics but not non-asthmatics is the purine nucleoside called adenosine. Bronchoconstriction is transient and probably mediated indirectly through a combination of mast cell-derived bronchoconstrictors and neural reflexes. Theophylline, in addition to other actions, antagonizes adenosine at the receptor level. There is little evidence at present that adenosine has a physiological role in asthma.

5.6.4 Complement

Complement is an integral part of the innate immune system and is composed of a number of plasma-derived protein mediators that have a range of pro-inflammatory activities. The system exists as inactive precursors that are enzymatically activated by an inflammatory insult to result in the generation of an amplified cascade of protein mediators in a manner similar to the clotting system. Two of the components of the system, the so-called 'anaphylotoxins' C3a and C5a, have been suggested to have a role in asthma because they are effective neutrophil and eosinophil chemoattractants, and in the skin at least, cause mast cell degranulation. Complement is activated in diseases characterized by immune complex deposition. However, there is no evidence for consumption of complement in asthma, and diseases such as systemic lupus erythematosis (SLE) that are known to involve complement have a very different clinical and pathological profile to asthma. Current evidence suggests that neither immune complexes nor complement components play a major part in asthma pathogenesis.

5.6.5 Oxygen radicals

Activation of eosinophils, neutrophils and macrophages *in vitro* readily causes the generation of oxygen radicals. These include the superoxide ion

(O_2^-), H_2O_2 and hydroxyl radicals (OH^-). These are highly reactive molecules that can markedly potentiate the tissue-damaging effects of peroxidase enzymes such as eosinophil peroxidase. Again their role in asthma remains speculative.

5.7 Summary and conclusions

As can be seen, many mediators have been implicated in playing a role in asthma. These can be loosely divided into mediators that cause bronchoconstriction, increased vascular permeability and mucus hypersecretion, mediators that cause leukocyte accumulation and mediators that cause epithelial damage. The criteria to establish if a mediator is likely to have a role in a disease process are detailed in *Table 5.2*. How well the mediators discussed in this chapter fit these criteria is outlined in *Table 5.13*. The evidence for most remains patchy. However, as will be seen in Chapter 7, this is an area of intense pharmacological activity, and a large number of antagonists will be available in the near future to test fully the hypothesis that the mediators discussed above play a role in the pathogenesis of asthma.

Table 5.13: Summary of mediators in asthma

Mediator	Major relevant activity	Increased in asthma (or allergen challenge)	Specific inhibitors effective
Histamine	Bronchoconstriction	Yes	No
$LTC_4/D_4/E_4$	Bronchoconstriction Mucus hypersecretion	Yes	Early studies suggest yes
PGD_2	Bronchoconstriction	Yes	No
PAF	Bronchoconstriction Leukocyte recruitment	No	Early studies suggest no
Neuropeptides	Bronchoconstriction	No	Not known
Kinins	Bronchoconstriction	Yes	Not known
LTB_4	Leukocyte recruitment	No	Not known
IL-4	IgE synthesis Th2-cell activation Eosinophil recruitment	Yes	Not known
IL-5	Eosinophil recruitment	Yes	Not known
RANTES	Eosinophil and lymphocyte recruitment	Not known	Not known
Complement	Leukocyte recruitment	No	Not known
Eosinophil granule proteins (e.g. MBP)	Epithelial damage	Yes	Not known
Oxygen radicals	Epithelial damage	No	Anti-oxidants ineffective

Further reading

Inflammatory mediators: general principles and reviews

Arm, J.P. and Lee, T.H. (1992) The pathobiology of bronchial asthma. *Adv. Immunol.,* **51**, 323–382.

Clemens, M.J. (1991) *Cytokines.* BIOS Scientific Publishers, Oxford.

Dale, M. and Foreman, J.C. (1993) *Textbook of Immunopharmacology,* 3rd Edn. Blackwell Scientific Publications, Oxford,

Holgate, S.T. (1993) Mediator and cytokine mechanisms in asthma. *Thorax,* **48**, 103–109.

Eosinophil granule proteins

Ackerman, S.J. (1993) Characterization and function of eosinophil granule proteins. in *Eosinophils, Biological and Clinical Aspects* (S. Makino and T. Fukuda, Eds). CRC Press, Boca Raton, pp. 33–74.

Filley, W.V., Holley, K.E., Kephart, G.M. and Gleich, G.J. (1982) Identification by immunofluorescence of eosinophil granule major basic protein in lung tissues of patients with bronchial asthma. *Lancet,* **2**, 11.

Gleich, G.J. and Adolphson, C.R. (1986) The eosinophil leukocyte: structure and function. *Adv. Immunol.,* **39**, 177–253.

Gundel, R.H., Letts, L.G. and Gleich, G.J. (1991) Human eosinophil major basic protein induces airway constriction and airway hyperresponsiveness in primates. *J. Clin. Invest.,* **87**, 1470.

Tai, P.C., Spry, C.J., Peterson, C., Venge, P. and Olssen, I. (1984) Monoclonal antibodies distinguish between storage and secreted forms of eosinophil cationic protein. *Nature,* **309**, 182.

Venge, P. (1993) Human eosinophil granule proteins. in *Immunopharmacology of Eosinophils* (H. Smith and R.M. Cook, Eds). Academic Press, New York, pp. 43–56.

Wardlaw, A.J., Dunnette, S., Gleich, G.J., Collins, J.V. and Kay, A.B. (1988) Eosinophils and mast cells in bronchoalveolar lavage in subjects with mild asthma: relationship to bronchial hyperreactivity. *Am. Rev. Respir. Dis.,* **137**, 62.

Histamine

Casale, T.B., Wood, D. and Richerson, H.B. *et al.* (1987) Elevated bronchoalveolar lavage fluid histamine levels in allergic asthmatics are associated with methacholine bronchial hyperresponsiveness. *J. Clin. Invest.,* **79**, 1197–1203.

Durham, S.R., Lee, T.H. and Cromwell, O. *et al.* (1984) Immunologic studies in allergen-induced late phase asthmatic reactions. *J. Allergy Clin. Immunol.,* **74**, 49–60.

Eiser, N.M., Mills, J., Snashall, P.D. and Guz, A. (1981) The role of histamine receptors in asthma. *Clin. Sci.,* **60**, 363–370.

Leukotrienes

Dahlen, S.-E., Hedqvist, P., Hammarstrom, S. and Samuelsson, B. (1980) Leukotrienes are potent constrictors of human bronchi. *Nature,* **288,** 481–486.

Ford Hutchinson, A.W., Bray, M.A., Doig, M.V., Shipley, M.E. and Smith, M.J.H. (1980) Leukotriene B, a potent chemokinetic and aggregating substance released from polymorphonuclear leucocytes. *Nature,* **286,** 264–265.

Marom, Z., Shelhamer, J.H., Bach, M.K., Morton, D.R. and Kaliner, M. (1982) Slow-reacting substances leukotrienes C4 and D4 increase the release of mucus from human airways *in vitro. Am. Rev. Respir. Dis.,* **126,** 449–451.

Miller, D.K., Gillard, J.W. and Vickers, P.J. *et al.* (1990) Identification and isolation of a membrane protein necessary for leukotriene production. *Nature,* **343,** 278–281.

O'Hickey, S.P., Hawksworth, R.J., Fong, C.Y., Arm, J.P., Spur, B.W. and Lee, T.H. (1991) Leukotrienes C4, D4 and E4 enhance histamine responsiveness in asthmatic airways. *Am. Rev. Respir. Dis.,* **144,** 1053–1057.

Rouzer, C.A., Rands, E. and Kargman, S. *et al.* (1988) Characterization of cloned human leukocyte 5-lipoxygenase expressed in mammalian cells. *J. Biol. Chem.,* **263,** 10135–10140.

Samuelsson, B. (1983) Leukotrienes: mediators of hypersensitvity reactions and inflammation. *Science,* **220,** 568–575.

Wardlaw, A.J., Hay, H., Cromwell, O., Collins, J.V. and Kay, A.B. (1989) Leukotrienes LTC4 and LTB4 in bronchoalveolar lavage fluid in bronchial asthma and other respiratory diseases. *J. Allergy Clin. Immunol.,* **84,** 19–26.

Wenzel, S.E., Larsen, G.L., Johnston, K., Voelkel, N.F. and Westcott, J.Y. (1990) Elevated levels of leukotriene C4 in bronchoalveolar lavage fluid from atopic asthmatics after endobronchial allergen challenge. *Am. Rev. Respir. Dis.,* **142,** 112–119.

Prostaglandins

Hardy, C.C., Robinson, C., Tattersfield, A.E. and Holgate, S.T. (1984) The bronchoconstrictor effect of inhaled prostaglandin D2 in normal and asthmatic men. *New Engl. J. Med.,* **311,** 209–313.

Lui, M.C., Bleeker, E.R. and Lichenstein, L.M. *et al.* (1990) Evidence for elevated levels of histamine, prostaglandin D2 and other bronchoconstricting prostaglandins in the airways of subjects with mild asthma. *Am. Rev. Respir. Dis.,* **142,** 126–132.

Samuelsson, B., Goldyne, M. and Granstrom, E. *et al.* (1978) Prostaglandins and thromboxanes. *Annu. Rev. Biochem.,* **47,** 997–1029.

Uotila, P. and Vapaatalo, H. (1984) Synthesis, pathways and biological implications of eicosanoids. *Ann. Clin. Res.,* **16,** 226–233.

Platelet-activating factor

Barnes, P.J. (1991) Inflammatory activities. *Nature,* **349,** 284–285.

Cuss, F.M., Dixon, C.M.S. and Barnes, P.J. (1986) Effects of platelet-activating factor on pulmonary function and bronchial responsiveness in man. *Lancet,* **2,** 189–192.

Demopolous, C.A., Pinckard, R.N. and Hanahan, R.J. (1979) Platelet activating factor: Evidence for 1-*O*-alkyl-2-acetyl-*sn*-glyceryl-3-phosphorylcholine as the active component of platelet activating factor (a new class of lipid chemical mediators). *J. Biol. Chem.,* **254,** 9355–9358.

Henocq, A.E. and Vargaftig, B.B. (1988) Skin eosinophilia in atopic patients. *J. Allergy Clin. Immunol.,* **81,** 691–695.

Honda, Z.-I., Nakamura, M. and Miki, I. *et al.* (1991) Cloning by functional expression of platelet-activating factor receptor from guinea-pig lung. *Nature,* **349,** 342–346.

Lai, L.K.W., Jenkins, J.R., Polosa, R. and Holgate, S.T. (1990) Inhaled PAF fails to induce airway hyperresponsiveness in normal human subjects. *J. Appl. Physiol.,* **68,** 919–926.

Rubin, A.-H.E., Smith, I.J. and Patterson, R. (1987) The bronchoconstrictor properties of platelet activating factor in humans. *Am. Rev. Respir. Dis.,* **136,** 1145–1151.

Synder, F. (1985) Chemical and biochemical aspects of platelet activating factor: a novel class of acetylated ether-linked choline phospholipids. *Med. Res. Rev.,* **5,** 107–140.

Wardlaw, A.J., Moqbel, R., Cromwell, O. and Kay, A.B. (1986) Platelet activating factor. A potent chemotactic and chemokinetic factor for human eosinophils. *J. Clin. Invest.,* **78,** 1701–1706.

Cytokines and cytokine receptors

Kameyoshi, Y., Dorschner, A., Mallet, A.I., Christophers, E. and Schroder, J.-M. (1992) Cytokine RANTES released by thrombin stimulated platelets is a potent attractant for human eosinophils. *J. Exp. Med.,* **176,** 587–592.

Kinashi, T., Harada, N. and Severinson, E. *et al.* (1986) Cloning of a complementary DNA encoding T cell replacing factor and identity with B cell growth factor. II. *Nature,* **324,** 70.

Miyajima, A., Kitamura, T., Harada, N., Yokota, T. and Arai, K.-I. (1992) Cytokine receptors and signal transduction. *Annu. Rev. Immunol.,* **10,** 295–331.

Murata, Y., Takaki, S. and Migita, M. *et al.* (1992) Molecular cloning and expression of the human interleukin 5 receptor. *J. Exp. Med.,* **175,** 341–351.

Neote, K., DiGregorio, D., Mak, J.Y., Horuk, R. and Schall, T. (1993) Molecular cloning, functional expression and signaling characteristics of a C-C chemokine receptor. *Cell,* **72,** 415–425.

Oppenheim, J.J., Zachariae, O., Mukaida, N. and Matsushima, K. (1991) Properties of the novel pro-inflammatory supergene "intercrine cytokine family". *Annu. Rev. Immunol.,* **9,** 617–648.

Robinson, D.S. (1993) Interleukin-5, eosinophils and bronchial hyperreactivity. *Clin. Exp. Allergy,* **23,** 1–3.

Sanderson, C.J., Campbell, H.D. and Young, I.G. (1988) Molecular and cellular biology of eosinophil differentiation factor (interleukin-5) and its effect on human and mouse B cells. *Immunol. Rev.*, **102**, 29.

Schall, T.J. (1991) Biology of the RANTES/SIS cytokine family. *Cytokine*, **3**, 165–183.

Van-Leeuwen, B.H., Martinson, M.E., Webb, G.C. and Young, I.G. (1989) Molecular organization of the cytokine gene cluster involving the human IL-3, IL-4, IL-5 and GM-CSF genes on human chromosome 5. *Blood*, **73**, 1142.

Walker, C., Virchow, J.-C., Bruijnzeel, P.L.B. and Blaser, K. (1991) T cell subsets and their soluble products regulate eosinophilia in allergic and non-allergic asthma. *J. Immunol.*, **146**, 1829–1835.

Chapter 6

The genetics of asthma

6.1 Introduction

Clinicians and patients have long recognized that asthma runs in families. Anecdotal observations have been supported by twin studies and family studies, which have suggested a multigene pattern of inheritance. This would fit with the multifactorial nature of asthma. The model of asthma pathogenesis advanced in this book proposes that an inhaled antigen sets up a specific T-lymphocyte/eosinophil mediated inflammatory response in the bronchi which, in individuals with susceptible airways, leads to asthma. This implies at least two levels of genetic control, one to determine the nature of the inflammatory response and the other to determine airways susceptibility. Moreover, control of the inflammatory response could have several genetic determinants: a gene(s) to determine a Th2 response to antigen, a gene(s) to determine IgE responsiveness and the degree of eosinophilia and a gene(s) to control the resolution of inflammation. Airway susceptibility remains a hazy concept, with only bronchial hyperresponsiveness representing a possible phenotype, and could be under the control of one or more genes (*Figure 6.1*).

This chapter summarizes the studies that have suggested a familial pattern of inheritance for asthma and bronchial hyperresponsiveness, discusses the recent studies that have pointed to a single gene on chromosome 11 for IgE responsiveness, and outlines the work done to characterize allergens and their interaction with the MHC and the T-cell receptor. Before describing this work a brief outline is given of some of the principles that underlie human genetics.

6.2 Basic principles of human genetics

Every nucleated cell in the human body contains 23 chromosomes, which are paired, making 46 chromosomes in total. One non-identical pair, the X and Y chromosomes, is involved in sex determination, leaving 44 autosomal chromosomes. Near the mid-point of each chromosome is a

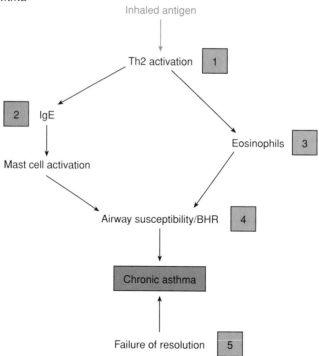

Figure 6.1: Schematic outline of the pathogenesis of asthma, indicating the various points at which genetic control may be important. (1) Determination of a specific type (Th2) of T-lymphocyte response to allergens possibly resulting from the nature of MHC haplotype, T-cell antigen receptor structure or other as yet undetermined factors. (2) Control of specific and total IgE production by B cells. (3) Control of the production and localization to the airways of eosinophils and other inflammatory cells. (4) Control of bronchial hyperresponsiveness. (5) Control of the events involved in resolution of the inflammatory process.

structure called a centromere, which is involved in partitioning of the chromosome during cell division.

The genetic material on each chromosome is composed of a double strand of DNA, containing the nucleosides deoxyadenosine (A), deoxycytidine (C), deoxythymine (T) and deoxyguanosine (G). A can pair with T, and C with G, by hydrogen bonding so that the two DNA strands are complementary (*Figures 6.2 and 6.3*). Individual nucleotides in a strand are joined by phosphodiester bonds, with the 5′-carbon of the deoxyribose moiety joining to the 3′-carbon of the adjacent nucleotide via the phosphate group (*Figure 6.4*).

Cells are able to convert the nucleotide sequence of a segment of a DNA molecule (a gene) into the amino acid sequence of a protein. They do this by first making an RNA copy of one strand of the DNA, a process called transcription. An RNA strand is slightly different from a DNA strand, as uracil is used instead of thymine (still pairing with adenine) and the sugar group is ribose instead of deoxyribose. The transcript is called

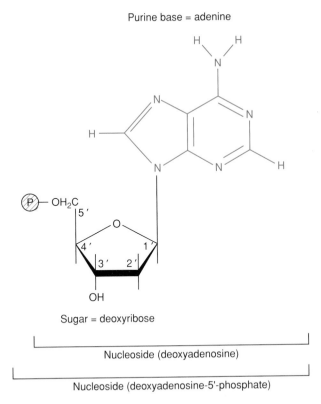

Purine base = adenine

Sugar = deoxyribose

Nucleoside (deoxyadenosine)

Nucleoside (deoxyadenosine-5'-phosphate)

Figure 6.2: Nucleotides, the building blocks of DNA, are composed of a purine (adenine or guanine) or pyrimidine (thymine or cytosine) base attached to a sugar moiety, 2'-deoxyribose, which has a phosphate group attached. In RNA the pyrimidine base uracil (U) is substituted for thymine and the sugar is ribose, in which a hydroxyl (OH) group is attached to the 2'-C position.

messenger ribonucleic acid (mRNA) and is transported from the nucleus of the cell to the cytoplasm, where the protein encoded by the mRNA is synthesized (a process called translation) on structures called ribosomes, many of which are attached to the endoplasmic reticulum (*Figure 6.5*).

Some cells make an enzyme that can reverse transcribe DNA from RNA. These reverse transcriptase enzymes have been invaluable in techniques in the molecular cloning of genes.

The location of a gene on a chromosome is called a locus. The key to the way in which the cell can read the gene to make the protein encoded by it is based on the genetic code, which is a triplet code. Each triplet of nucleotides represents a single amino acid. With four nucleotides there are 64 potential triplet combinations. As there are only 20 amino acids this means that the code is degenerate (i.e. more than one triplet codes for most individual amino acids).

Many genes in humans, as in all eukaryotic organisms, are not a single continuous section of DNA, but are divided into a number of discrete

(a)

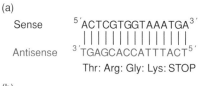

Thr: Arg: Gly: Lys: STOP

(b)

Adenine   Thymine
                 N

Guanine   Cytosine

Figure 6.3: The double helix structure of DNA consists of two chains of nucleotides linked by hydrogen bonds between complementary bases: adenine pairs with thymine, and guanine with cytosine (b). Regions of DNA that are transcribed into RNA are called genes; many of these genes code for proteins. The genetic code specifies the nucleotide triplets that code for individual amino acids. In the example given (a) a sequence of 15 nucleotides codes for threonine, arginine, glycine, lysine, followed by a codon which specifies the end of the polypeptide chain.

units (exons) that are separated by regions of DNA which do not code for protein (introns). The introns are removed (spliced out) after the mRNA strand is made. Introns are often much larger than exons, so that a gene whose coding regions total 2 kb may span a region of chromosomal DNA which is tens of kb in length. Expression of genes is controlled by various regulatory elements, including regions that promote or repress transcription.

The simplest types of genetic disorder are those in which a single gene is mutated, as occurs with cystic fibrosis (CF). However, even with a single-gene disorder, in unrelated individuals with the disease there may be many different types of mutation affecting different regions of the gene. These can include deleted regions of DNA, insertions of new sequences of nucleotides, or single-nucleotide mutations that alter the amino acid coded by a triplet. The mutations may completely inhibit the protein synthesis or may merely impair the function of the protein, so that it works, but not in the correct way or with the normal degree of activity. In

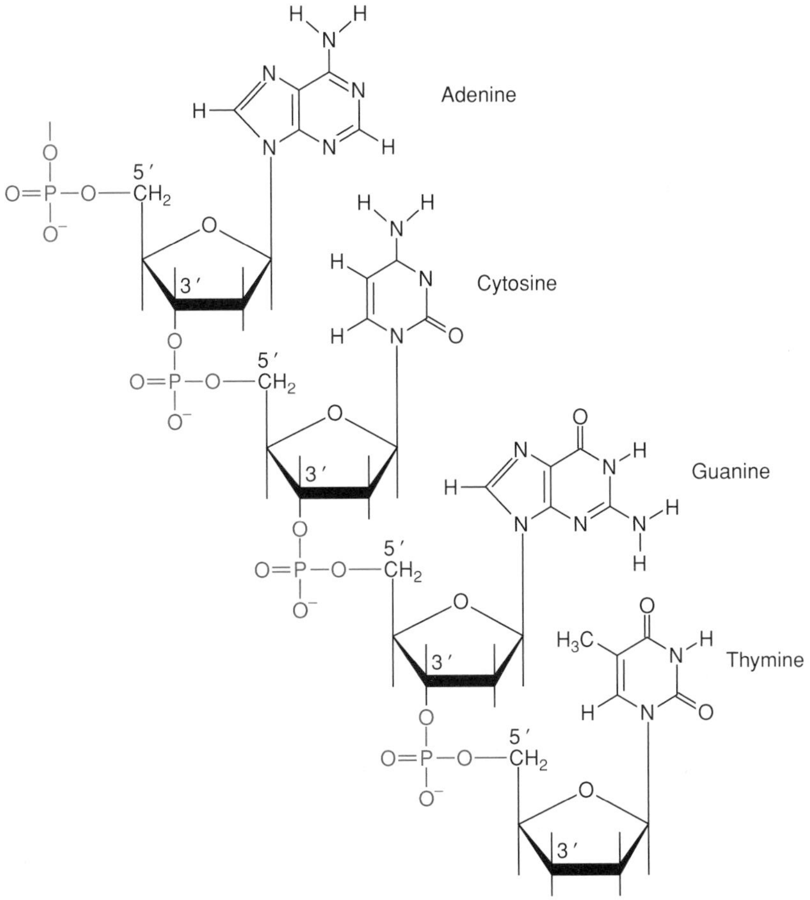

Figure 6.4: In a DNA strand, adjacent nucleotides are linked by phosphodiester bonds between 5'- and 3'-carbons.

the former case the disease resulting from complete lack of the protein may be severe, whereas in the latter case it may be mild. Even in single-gene disorders such as CF, patients with the same mutation may have varying severity of disease, emphasizing the importance of environmental effects and interactions with other genes.

Mutations can occur randomly when the cell divides as a result of errors in DNA replication. Some regions of DNA (hypervariable regions) are more prone to mutations than other regions. In a non-germline cell a mutation is called somatic and its effects are limited to that cell and to its progeny. Generally, the result will be unremarkable, although malignant cells can result from this process. However, if the DNA in the sperm or egg mutates, then the error will be passed to the embryo, and every cell in the fetus will be mutated. This mutation may result in a situation in which the embryo cannot develop and a miscarriage will result, or it may be silent and not be noticed so that the appearance (phenotype) of the child

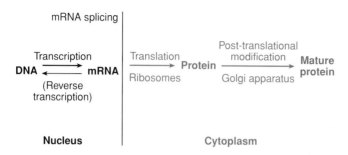

Figure 6.5: Protein coding genes are transcribed into messenger RNA. This initially is a copy of the gene comprising both non-protein coding regions (introns) and coding regions (exons). The introns are spliced out and the mRNA then transported to ribosomes in the cytoplasm, where the protein chain is constructed. The protein chain can be modified in a number of ways, for example by the addition of sugar groups or by cleavage into smaller chains.

will not be different despite the mutated genotype, or it may alter the activity of a protein, resulting in a change in the phenotype of the child. This may be a subtle change, such as a different eye color, or a pronounced difference leading to disease.

As we have two of each chromosome, inheriting one from each parent, we have two genes for each protein. In many disease conditions both genes need to be abnormal before the disease is manifested: these are called recessive diseases (autosomal recessive if the gene is not sex linked). If an abnormality in only one of the genes can cause disease, then the condition is said to be dominant. Whether a disease is dominant or recessive can be determined from the pattern of inheritance, as recessive genes may be silent in the parents, whereas dominant genes are always expressed (*Figure 6.6*). If a phenotype (for example blood pressure) has a normal distribution in a population then it can generally be concluded that it is under the control of a number of genes, as single-gene disorders are usually characterized by a bimodal (yes or no) distribution.

Genes are rarely identical in two individuals or even on chromosomes in the same individual, containing at least one or two base pair differences. These are called polymorphisms. Many such differences either do not change the amino acid that is specified or result in the substitution of a similar amino acid whose insertion does not affect the function of the protein.

6.2.1 Reverse genetics

An important feature of chromosome activity is a process called crossing over. This occurs during meiosis when the germ cells are formed. During meiosis each chromosome divides into two chromatids, and paired chromosomes come together and coil around each other. Breaks occur in the chromosomes, and can rejoin to the other chromosome in the pair rather than to the original chromosome. In this way genetic material can be transferred between chromosomes.

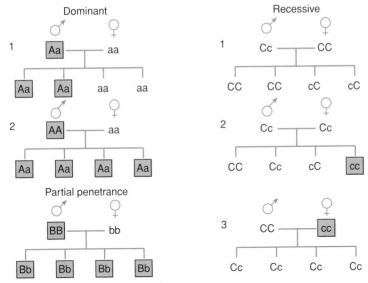

Figure 6.6: Single-gene patterns of disease inheritance. In the dominant example the disease is carried by the 'A' allele and the presence of disease in an individual is indicated by heavy shading. If, as in example 1, one of the four alleles involved carries the disease, 50% of the offspring will be affected, whereas if two or more alleles are affected (example 2), from either parent, all offspring will have the disease. An example of this type of disease is Huntington's chorea. In the recessive example, corresponding to a disease such as cystic fibrosis, the disease is carried by the allele 'c'. Disease can occur only if both parents have the allele.

If two genes lie close together on the same chromosome then they are said to be linked, as they will tend to stay together during crossing over. If they are further apart they will be less likely to stay together (*Figure 6.7*). The degree of linkage displayed by two genes gives an approximate measure of the physical distance between them on the chromosome. This is the basis of the process called reverse genetics, which has been used with great success to identify the genes responsible for a number of inherited disorders.

In reverse genetics an attempt is made to find linkage between a region of DNA of known location and the phenotype which represents the disease. The more clearly defined the phenotype, the greater the likelihood of success. A variety of DNA analysis techniques can be used in conjunction with pedigree studies to identify a region of DNA that is linked to the disease gene. This linked region is then used as the starting point for a cloning program that will hopefully isolate the disease gene. Some genes which have been discovered using this approach are listed in *Table 6.1*.

6.3 Family and twin studies in asthma

Family studies in the 1950s and 1960s demonstrated an increased prevalence of asthma and allergic disease in first-degree relatives of

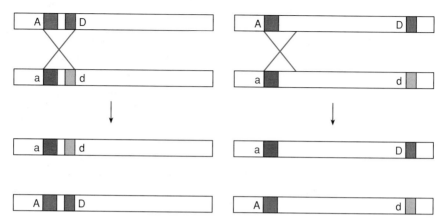

Figure 6.7: Linkage of physically related areas of DNA during crossing over. In this example the disease is carried by the 'd' allele, with 'D' being the normal or 'wild-type' allele. The regions A and a are two unrelated alleles corresponding to a known region of DNA. This could represent a gene with a known function such as eye color, where 'A' might represent blue eyes and 'a' brown eyes, or merely a region of the chromosome identified through use of a DNA probe. In the left-hand example the disease gene is physically close to the A region on the chromosome, so that when crossing over occurs during meiosis the two regions are likely to stay together. In the case where A and a represent eye color, the disease allele 'd' would be linked to brown eyes and the wild-type allele to blue eyes. In the right-hand example the disease gene is not closely linked to the A region and is much more likely to become separated as a result of crossing over. In this case there will be no clear linkage between eye color and the disease.

Table 6.1: Disease genes isolated by reverse genetics

Duchenne muscular dystrophy
Myotonic dystrophy
Cystic fibrosis
Neurofibromatosis
Chronic granulomatous disease
Retinoblastoma

sufferers compared with the general population. This finding was also supported by twin studies, in which the prevalence of asthma is compared in monozygotic (genetically identical twins derived from the same fertilized egg) and dizygotic twins derived from different eggs. In both types of twins environmental stimuli are considered to be broadly the same, so that differences in the degree of concordance (i.e. when both twins have asthma) between di- and monozygotic twins are regarded as a measure of the importance of genetic influences on the disease.

A large study by Edfors-Lubs in 1971 of 7000 twins revealed a concordance of 19% in monozygotic twins and 5% in dizygotic twins.

More recent studies have shown an even greater difference between the two types of twins, implying a greater degree of heritability. Twin studies, while providing evidence of a genetic involvement, tell us nothing about the mode of inheritance; for this, family studies are necessary.

Families can be either nuclear, consisting only of first-degree relatives, or extended, in which case more distant relations are included. Large extended families are often more useful in determining hereditary patterns but may have a gene mutation which is unrepresentative of that which is usually present in the disease or phenotype in question. Nuclear families are often easier to recruit.

Family studies start with an affected individual called a proband. How the proband is recruited is important, as it may introduce attainment bias, which means that the sample of the population studied is unrepresentative of the disease in the whole population. A number of family studies of asthma have been performed and have consistently demonstrated an increased prevalence of asthma among relatives of extrinsic asthmatics compared with controls, about 10% compared with 2%. Studies of intrinsic asthma have been more variable but have generally shown an increased prevalence. In one recent study, 8% of siblings of intrinsic asthmatics had asthma compared with 2.4% of non-asthmatic controls. Despite this evidence for a familial component to asthma, no clear pattern of inheritance has emerged, with some studies suggesting an autosomal dominant pattern with incomplete penetrance and other commentators suggesting a polygenic inheritance. The lack of a clear-cut picture with asthma taken as a whole has led investigators to study individual aspects of the asthma diathesis, including control of IgE, bronchial hyperresponsiveness and response to allergens.

6.4 Genetics of bronchial hyperresponsiveness

Bronchial hyperresponsiveness (BHR) is still an ill-understood phenomenon. It is clearly associated with airways inflammation, and there is increasing evidence that in asthma it may be the result of thickening of the bronchial wall (see Chapter 2). In the general population there is a unimodal (normal) distribution in the response to bronchoconstrictors such as histamine and methacholine. This is generally regarded as suggesting a polygenic pattern of inheritance, although a single gene with variable penetrance could also be consistent with a normally distributed phenotype.

There is some evidence to suggest that the degree of responsiveness of the airways to non-specific irritants, although related to asthma and influenced by airways inflammation, is under independent control which includes a genetic component. For example, within an asthmatic population the degree of BHR does not correlate with the airways eosinophilia. In population studies about 5% of individuals without a history of asthma have a Pc20 that falls into the asthmatic range. Twin studies of BHR demonstrate an increased concordance in monozygotic twins and there is an increased incidence of BHR in non-asthmatic parents of asthmatic children compared with the normal population.

Animal studies also support a genetic basis for BHR, in that inbred strains of mice and rats can show markedly different BHR between strains. In one study of Brown Norway rats hyperresponsiveness to 5-hydroxytryptamine had a recessive pattern of inheritance. A clear understanding of the extent to which BHR is genetically controlled probably awaits a fuller understanding of its pathogenesis.

6.5 Genetics of IgE responsiveness

6.5.1 General considerations

The close association between asthma and atopy has led to intense investigation into the reasons why some people produce IgE in large amounts and others only in small amounts. There are two ways to consider IgE: total serum IgE and IgE specific to allergens. Even in atopic individuals most serum IgE is directed against unknown antigens and not the commonly recognized allergens. Extrinsic asthma and other allergic diseases are clinically associated with the presence of specific IgE, as evidenced by positive skin prick test reactions and RAST tests, rather than high levels of total IgE *per se*.

As discussed in Chapter 3, IgE is produced when B cells encounter antigen in concert with a membrane stimulus from helper T cells and IL-4. This is a complex process with several different levels of control, some of which will determine the amount of IgE produced for a given stimulus and others, such as the nature of the stimulus, determining whether IgE is produced, rather than another Ig isotype. Theoretically at least, total IgE and specific IgE could be under the control of a related but distinct set of factors. It should be remembered that most individuals can make IgE in large amounts under certain circumstances. For example, in areas where infection with helminthic parasites is endemic, such parasites stimulate a vigorous IgE response. There is no evidence that asthma is more common in these areas; indeed it often appears to be less common.

These considerations are of more than arcane interest because they determine the phenotype (either total IgE or specific IgE (atopy)) that will be used in genetic studies, and much of the debate regarding the genetics of IgE has been focused around the question of the phenotype chosen. In Britain, where infection with IgE-producing parasites is rare, increased amounts of total IgE and the presence of atopy may be expected to converge, although high levels of endemic infections with potentially IgE-stimulating parasites such as *Toxocara canis* may confound matters. One problem with measurement of IgE is that it decreases with age, and methods to adjust for this are only approximations. In addition, recent allergen exposure may complicate the issue, so studies should be performed outside the pollen season.

6.5.2 Twin and family studies

Studies have shown increased concordance for total IgE production in monozygotic compared with dizygotic twins. A number of population studies have been performed in attempts to determine the pattern of inheritance of IgE levels, but no entirely consistent picture has emerged. On average, the importance of heritability in determination of IgE serum levels has been estimated to be 50%. Early studies with nuclear families suggested a recessive pattern of inheritance for high IgE, but pedigree studies have suggested heterogeneity, with some pedigrees having a dominant pattern for high IgE, and others recessive or mixed. One study investigated 42 nuclear families with a total of 278 individuals recruited through employment for Westinghouse Corporation in Baltimore. When adjusting for sex and age and taking blood outside the pollen season, segregation analysis best fitted a recessive mode of inheritance for high IgE. In summary, therefore, it seems clear that total IgE levels in the blood are determined to a considerable extent by genetic factors. Whether there is a single gene or whether inheritance is polygenic cannot be determined with any certainty, although the majority of studies have suggested a single recessive gene. However, there seems to be considerable genetic heterogeneity between families.

6.5.3 IgE and chromosome 11q

For the reasons discussed above, most studies have tended to investigate specific and total IgE as if they were separately determined. However, one group, directed by Cookson and Hopkin in Oxford, UK, took a different approach. The phenotype they studied was much broader, involving any evidence of increased IgE responsiveness. Thus they regarded someone as atopic if they displayed a wheal of 2 mm greater than the control on skin prick testing to a range of common allergens, and/or had raised total IgE, and/or had an increased RAST. Using this all-inclusive definition they obtained evidence of an autosomal dominant pattern of inheritance. They went on to see if they could obtain linkage between their atopic phenotype and a region of DNA using the methods of reverse genetics. They analyzed genomic DNA digested with the restriction enzyme *TaqI* using DNA probes from various regions of the genome. By using probes which represent regions of the genome that are highly polymorphic (i.e. have a high rate of mutation and therefore give a different pattern of bands between most individuals) they found that one probe representing a region of DNA on chromosome 11 called MS.51 (now called D11S97), gave a pattern of bands that coincided with affected individuals. This was particularly striking in one extended family (*Figure 6.8*). This pattern was seen in four out of six extended families and was confirmed in 64 two-generation nuclear families.

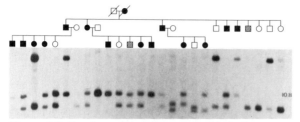

Figure 6.8: Southern blot of genomic DNA from an extended family with a high incidence of atopy probed with a DNA marker from a known region of chromosome 11q. The filled symbols represent the presence of atopy. In nearly all individuals the presence of atopy corresponds to a 10.8 kb restriction fragment. Reprinted from Cookson *et al.* (1989) with permission from *The Lancet*.

This linkage to chromosome 11 is only seen in alleles derived from the maternal side, which supports the observation that the risk of atopy is greater when the mother rather than the father is atopic, and accounts for atopy in about 60% of the families that have been studied. The lod scores obtained by this group are very high, ruling out a chance observation. A number of groups have failed to replicate this observation using similar methodology with both nuclear family and pedigree studies and using probands with asthma, rhinitis and atopic dermatitis. However, the numbers of individuals studied by other groups have tended to be small or the patients have been from different ethnic groups, which may be relevant if there is genetic heterogeneity. Although this lack of confirmation is disappointing, linkage analysis is complex, and some variability in findings is to be expected. The Oxford group's data are convincing. The key question is whether they can use their findings to locate the putative gene with which they have linkage. Two candidate genes in the region of chromosome 11 where the atopic gene was localized (region 11q13) are CD20 and the gene for the β-chain of the high-affinity Fc IgE receptor (Chapter 4). There is an obvious, although indirect, connection between the IgE receptor on mast cells and atopy, making this a possible candidate for the 'atopy gene' suggested by these workers.

6.6 Structure of allergens

Asthma and related allergic diseases are unusual among the chronic inflammatory diseases in that the nature of the antigen that initiated the disease process can sometimes be identified. Furthermore, the type of immune response elicited by these antigens, being associated with IgE synthesis and an eosinophilia, is of a very specific type. It was therefore hoped that characterization of the proteins involved would lead to an understanding of what makes an antigen an allergen.

As detailed in Chapter 1, allergens are proteins usually derived from plant pollens, fungal spores, animal danders or excreta, certain foods and the venom of wasps and bees. Sensitization is usually across the mucosal surfaces of the gastrointestinal or respiratory tract or through the skin. As discussed in Chapter 3, antigens bind directly to the B-cell antigen receptor, whereas T cells interact with antigen only after it has been processed into peptide fragments by antigen-presenting cells. B cells therefore recognize the whole antigen and recognition is dependent on its three-dimensional structure. In contrast, T cells will respond to oligopeptide fragments of the antigen.

The regions (epitopes) of an antigen recognized by B cells and T cells are often different. Any one source of an allergen, such as the fecal pellet of the house dust mite, may contain a number of allergenic proteins. If a protein stimulates an allergenic response in most atopic individuals it is regarded as a major allergen and if a response is seen in only a few individuals it is regarded as a minor allergen. Many allergens have now been fully characterized, including their nucleotide sequence. Several have enzymatic activity. For example, the honey bee major allergen (Api m 1) is a phospholipase A_2 enzyme that is related to phospholipase A_2 from other species. Some allergens are related to known proteins in other species, for example, the major allergen from house dust mite (Der P 1) is related to the cysteine protease cathepsin. However, there is no structure common to all allergens, and homologies with other proteins have not revealed any clues as to the basis of their allergenic nature. It is possible that a more detailed understanding of the three-dimensional structures of allergens may reveal hitherto unrecognized common structural motifs. However, T-cell recognition is independent of three-dimensional structure and it appears to be the T-cell signal, both physical and cytokine, that determines whether a B-cell isotype switches to make IgE.

As discussed below, the nature of the T-cell antigen receptor and class II HLA receptor haplotype may help determine whether an antigen produces an allergenic response. It is clear from animal models that the timing, amount and route of sensitization are crucial factors. This is supported by studies in children suggesting that it is the level of allergen in the home in infancy that is important in determining atopic status, rather than the level of allergen in later childhood. Characterization of allergens has allowed detailed analysis of the interaction between immune recognition and antigen structure. This may well facilitate the development of effective and safe vaccines for immunotherapy, but it has so far failed to shed any real light on the crucial question of what makes an antigen an allergen.

6.7 Asthma and the MHC

Immune recognition is based on antigen being presented to T lymphocytes, which through their T-cell receptors recognize specific antigens in combination with HLA receptors expressed by antigen-presenting cells. In particular, there is increasing evidence that the airways inflammation characterisitic of asthma in many cases is the result of the host responding to inhaled allergens by triggering of a specific subset of T-helper CD4+ve cells (Th2) cells, which generate IL-4 and IL-5. Complex antigens such as allergens are taken up by antigen-presenting cells (e.g. dendritic cells, airways macrophages and B lymphocytes) and then processed and presented to the T cell as an oligopeptide about 20 amino acids long bound to the floor of the groove that constitutes the structure of the HLA class II receptor.

An allergen can be broken down into a number of peptides that will provoke an immune response. Although any one allele of a class II receptor can bind a number of peptides there is a degree of restriction, with some alleles binding certain peptides more avidly than others. One hypothesis is that some people are more susceptible to a disease, particularly an autoimmune disease, because their genetically inherited HLA receptor alleles (their HLA haplotype) means that they can present certain antigens very readily, so provoking a vigorous and inappropriately directed T-cell response. Investigators have therefore looked for associations between disease and HLA haplotypes, and several have been found. For example, insulin-dependent diabetes mellitus (IDDM) is associated with DQβ and rheumatoid arthritis with DRβ1. The nucleotide sequences of the genes for the HLA proteins involved has been established and the mutations related to disease determined. For IDDM the absence of an aspartic acid on the DQβ chain at position 51 confers susceptibility.

HLA associations with specific IgE responses to allergen are variable, with clear associations to some simple allergens but not to larger, more complex, allergens. One of the closest associations has been found between the phenotype HLA-DR2.2 and production of specific IgE to the ragweed allergen Amb a V. In one study, 27 out of 29 subjects with an IgE response to Amb a V had the DR2.2 phenotype, whereas only 10 out of 56 negative controls had this phenotype. Further analysis of this association demonstrated that the ability of the HLA class II receptor represented by the DR2.2 phenotype to present Amb a V to T cells was due to neutral amino acids, as opposed to charged amino acids, being present in certain positions in the peptide-binding groove of the receptor. Looser associations have been found between other allergens and HLA haplotypes.

The lack of very tight associations between HLA haplotype and most allergens is perhaps not surprising given the complexity of allergens, which contain many different antigenic regions, and the redundancy of the HLA system, which by necessity can bind many different peptides, albeit with variable affinity. It seems therefore that, while HLA haplotype may modulate the degree and extent of an individual's atopic response, it is unlikely to be a deciding factor in whether or not a person is atopic.

6.8 T-cell receptor restriction and asthma

An individual who is to mount an immune response to allergen must have T cells with an antigen receptor specific for the allergen. As discussed in Chapter 3, the T-cell receptor is composed of an α- and β-chain, each with polymorphic regions, resulting in each T cell having a unique pattern of antigen recognition. In autoimmune disease there is some evidence that T cells at inflammatory sites have a restricted range of receptors, in particular in their use of the β-chain variable gene. They are oligoclonal, and instead of being derived from a large number of progenitor T cells are derived from a limited number, with similar T-cell receptors recognizing a similar antigen. Whether this is the case with asthma has not yet been determined. To do so will require airway T cells from asthmatics to be extracted and the structures of their antigen receptors determined. This will be complemented by *in vitro* studies analyzing the repertoire of T-cell clones to various allergenic epitopes.

6.9 Conclusion

In conclusion, asthma is likely to be the result of a specific inflammatory process interacting with a susceptible airway best defined at present as bronchial hyperresponsiveness. Genetic control of BHR may be distinct from those factors controlling the inflammatory process. Population and family studies of both intrinsic and extrinsic asthma have clearly demonstrated that genetic factors are important. Most work has focused on the genetics of the IgE response, partly because of the close association between atopy and asthma and partly because of the previous dominance of the mast cell hypothesis in our model of asthma pathogenesis. No definitive picture of the inheritability of IgE responsiveness has emerged, although the work of Cookson and Hopkin in Oxford, UK, offers the possibility of a major breakthrough in this area in the near future. More recently, the awareness of the importance of the T cell in asthma has led to studies on the relationship between asthma, allergen responsiveness and T cell–MHC interactions. This work is still in its early stages but offers great promise for the future.

Further reading

General

Anon (1990) Dissecting the complex diseases. *Science*, **247**, 1540–1542.

Blumenthal, M.N. and Amos, D.B. (1987) Genetic and immunologic basis of atopic diseases. *Chest*, **91**, 176S–184S.

Clinical and Experimental Allergy (1992) Volume 22. Much of this issue is taken up with articles on the likelihood of a major locus for IgE responsiveness.

Marsh, D.G., Lockhart, A. and Holgate, S.T. (Eds) (1993) *The Genetics of Asthma*. Blackwell Scientific Publications, Oxford.

Family and twin studies of asthma genetics

Edfors-Lubs, M.L. (1971) Allergy in 7000 twin pairs. *Acta Allergol.*, **26**, 249–285.

Gerrard, J., Vickers, P. and Gerrard, C. (1976) The familial incidence of allergic disease. *Ann. Allergy,* **36,** 10–15.

Hopp, R.J., Bewtra, A.K., Watt, G.D., Nair, N.M. and Townley, R.G. (1984) Genetic analysis of allergic disease in twins. *J. Allergy Clin. Immunol.,* **73,** 265–270.

Marsh, D., Meyers, D. and Bias, W. (1981) The epidemiology and genetics of atopic allergy. *New Engl. J. Med.,* **305,** 1551–1559.

Sibbald, B. and Turner-Warwick, M. (1979) Factors influencing the prevalence of asthma amongst first degree relatives of extrinsic and intrinsic asthmatics. *Thorax,* **34,** 332–337.

Sibbald, B., Horn, M., Brain, E. and Gregg, I. (1980) Genetic factors in childhood asthma. *Thorax,* **35,** 671–674.

Genetics of bronchial hyperresponsiveness

Pauwels, R., van der Straeten, M., Weyne, J. and Bazin, H. (1985) Genetic factors in non-specific bronchial reactivity in rats. *Eur. J. Respir. Dis.,* **66,** 98–104.

Townley, R.G., Bewtra, A., Wilson, A.F., Hopp, R.J., Elston, R.C., Nair, N. and Watt, G.D. (1986) Segregation analysis of bronchial response to methacholine inhalation challenge in families with and without asthma. *J. Allergy Clin. Immunol.,* **77,** 101–107.

Genetics of IgE

Blumenthal, M.N., Namboodiri, K., Mendell, N., Gleich, G., Elston, R.C. and Yunis, E. (1981) Genetic transmission of serum IgE levels. *Am. J. Genet.,* **10,** 219–228.

Blumenthal, M.N., Yunis, E., Mendell, N. and Elston, R.C. (1986) Preventive allergy: genetics of IgE mediated diseases. *J. Allergy Clin. Immunol.,* **78,** 962–968.

Burrows, B., Martinez, F.D., Halonen, M., Barbee, R.A. and Cline, M.G. (1989) Association of asthma with serum IgE levels and skin test reactivity to allergens. *New Engl. J. Med.,* **320,** 271–277.

Cookson, W.O.C.M. and Hopkin, J.M. (1988) Dominant inheritance of atopic immunoglobulin E responsiveness. *Lancet,* **1,** 86–88.

Cookson, W.O.C.M., Sharp, P.A., Faux, J.A. and Hopkin, J.M. (1989) Linkage between immunoglobulin E responses underlying asthma and rhinitis and chromosome 11q. *Lancet,* **1,** 1292–1295.

Gerrard, J.W., Rao, D.C. and Morton, N.E. (1978) A genetic study of immunoglobulin E. *Am. J. Hum. Genet.,* **30,** 46–58.

Hanson, B., McGue, M., Roitman-Johnson, B., Segal, N.L., Bouchard, T.J. Jr and Blumenthal, M.N. (1991) Atopic disease and immunoglobulin E in twins reared apart and together. *Am. J. Hum. Genet.,* **48,** 873–879.

Sandford, A.J., Shirakawa, T., Moffatt, M.F. *et al.* (1993) Localization of atopy and the β subunit of high affinity IgE-receptor (FcεR1) on chromosome 11q. *Lancet,* **341,** 332–334.

Atopy and the MHC

Blumenthal, M.N., Marcus-Bagley, D., Awdeh, Z., Johnson, B., Yunis, E.J. and Alper, C.A. (1992) HLA-DR2, (HLA-B7, SC31, DR2) and (HLA-B8, SC01, Dr3) haplotypes distinguish subjects with asthma from those with rhinitis only in ragweed pollen allergy. *J. Immunol.,* **148,** 411–416.

Huang, S.K., Zwollo, P. and Marsh, D.G. (1991) Class 2 MHC restriction of human T cell responses to short ragweed allergen Amb a V. *Eur. J. Immunol.,* **21,** 1469–1473.

Marsh, D.G. and Huang, S.K. (1991) Molecular genetics of human immune responsiveness to pollen allergens. *Clin. Exp. Allergy,* **21** (Suppl.), 1469–1473.

Marsh, D.G., Hsu, S.-H., Roebber, M., Ehrlich-Kautzky, E., Freidhoff, L.R., Meyers, D.A., Pollard, M.K. and Bias, W.B. (1982). HLA-Dw2: a genetic marker for human immune response to short ragweed pollen allergens Ra5. I. Response resulting primarily from natural antigenic exposure. *J. Exp. Med.,* **155,** 1439–1451.

O'Hehir, R.E., Mach, B., Berte, C., Greenlaw, R., Tiercy, J.M., Bal, V., Lechler, R.I., Trowsdale, J. and Lamb, J.R. (1990). Direct evidence for a functional role of HLA-DRB3 gene products in the recognition of *Dermatophagoides* spp. allergens by helper T-cell clones. *Int. Immunol.,* **2,** 885–892.

Allergenic structure

Chapman, M.D. (1991) Manipulating allergen genes. *Clin. Exp. Allergy,* **21,** 155–156.

Chua, K.Y., Dilworth, R.J. and Thomas, W.R. (1988) Sequence analysis of cDNA coding for a major house dust mite allergen. Der P 1. Homology with cysteine proteases. *J. Exp. Med.,* **167,** 175–182.

Schou, C. (1993) Defining allergens of mammalian origin. *Clin. Exp. Allergy,* **23,** 7–14.

Sprik, R., Holgate, S.T., Platts-Mills, T.A.E. and Cogswell, J.J. (1990) Exposure to house dust mite allergen (Der P 1) and the development of asthma in childhood: a prospective study. *New Engl. J. Med.,* **323,** 502–507.

T cells and allergens

O'Hehir, R.E., Garman, R.D., Greenstein, J.L. and Lamb, J.R. (1991) The specificity and T cell regulation of responsiveness to allergens. *Annu. Rev. Immunol.,* **9,** 76–95.

Chapter 7

Treatments for asthma, present and future

7.1 Introduction

The current understanding of asthma as a chronic inflammatory disease of the airways has led to a consensus that the appropriate treatment for asthma is a combination of regular anti-inflammatory medication to suppress the inflammatory response ('preventer medication'), and drugs used intermittently to reverse bronchospasm ('reliever medication'). These drugs are used in concert with a strategy to minimize exposure to both specific and non-specific asthma triggers. Currently two classes of anti-inflammatory drugs are in common use as preventer medications, disodium cromoglycate/nedocromil and glucocorticoids. Three classes of drugs are used routinely as reliever medications: β_2-agonists, anti-cholinergics and theophyllines (*Table 7.1*). However, as a result of the increased understanding of the pathogenesis of asthma described in the previous chapters, we are on the threshold of a new therapeutic era in which a range of novel medications will be designed to target the components of the inflammatory response in a more specific manner. The degree to which these are successful will depend on the extent to which current hypotheses about the nature of asthma are correct. Some of these approaches are outlined in *Table 7.2*. This chapter summarizes the basic pharmacology of the drugs currently used in asthma management and their likely mechanisms of action. In the second half of the chapter various new approaches being taken in asthma treatment will be described.

7.2 Current therapies for asthma: anti-inflammatory drugs

7.2.1 Glucocorticoids (corticosteroids)

Introduction. Glucocorticoids (GCs) are a family of four-carbon-ring, C_{21} steroids produced in the adrenal cortex from cholesterol through a

Table 7.1: Some drugs currently used in the treatment of asthma in the USA and Europe

Class of drug	Generic name	Trade name
(a) *'Preventers'*: anti-inflammatory drugs		
Glucocorticoids	Hydrocortisone (parenteral)	
	Prednisolone (oral)	
	Triamcinolone (parenteral, inhaled)	Azmacort
	Beclomethasone (inhaled)	Becatide/Beclaforte/Vanceril
	Budesonide (inhaled)	Pulmicort
	Flunisolide (inhaled)	Aerobid/Bronalide
	Betamethasone (oral, inhaled)	Bextasol
	Fluticasone (inhaled)	Flixatide
Non-steroid based	Disodium cromoglycate (inhaled)	Intal
	Nedocromil sodium (inhaled)	Tilade
(b) *'Relievers'*: bronchodilators		
β_2-Agonists	Salbutamol/albuterol	Ventolin
	Terbutaline	Bricanyl
	Pirbuterol	Maxair
	Bitolerol	Tornalate
	Fenoterol	Berotec
	Salmeterol	Serevent
	Formoterol	
Anti-cholinergics	Ipratropium bromide	Atrovent
	Oxitropium bromide	Oxivent
Phosphodiesterase inhibitors/adenosine antagonists	Theophylline/aminophylline	Phyllocontin Nuelin/many others

Table 7.2: New approaches to the treatment of asthma

Approach	Example
1. Modifications of existing treatment	Glucocorticoids with better side-effect profile
	Immunosuppressants with better side-effects
	Longer acting β_2-agonists (e.g. salmeterol)
	More specific phosphodiesterase inhibitors
	Anti-cholinergics targeted against the M3 receptor
2. Mediator antagonists	Leukotriene antagonists/synthesis inhibitors
	PAF antagonists/synthesis inhibitors
	Cytokine antagonists (anti-IL-5, anti-IL-4)
3. Immunomodulation	Immunotherapy with more specific allergens or peptide fragments to desensitize atopic individuals
	Induction of anergy or Th2 to Th1 switching in T-cell response to allergens
5. Anti-adhesion molecules	Antibodies against ICAM-1,VLA-4,VCAM-1
	Modification of carbohydrate metabolism to interfere with selectin receptor function
4. Cytokines	Interferon-γ/α

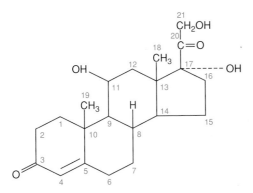

Figure 7.1: Structure of the naturally occurring glucocorticoid cortisol showing the four carbon rings and the ordering of the 21 carbons that make up the cortisol backbone.

complex biosynthetic cascade that results in the production of cortisol (hydrocortisone) and cortisone, the two naturally occurring glucocorticoids (*Figure 7.1*). Glucocorticoid secretion is controlled by production of adrenocorticotrophic hormone (ACTH) in the pituitary gland, which in turn is controlled by neurally stimulated secretion of corticotrophin-releasing factor (CRF) from the hypothalamus. Glucocorticoid levels control ACTH secretion by negative feedback.

Glucocorticoids have an important physiological role controlling carbohydrate and protein metabolism and the response to bodily stress. The importance of glucocorticoids is illustrated by the deficiency state Addison's disease, which results from destruction of the adrenal gland by tuberculosis, metastatic malignant disease or autoimmune disease. This results in dehydration, low blood glucose, hypotension and lethargy. In its severe form it can cause collapse and death. Addison's disease is due to a combination of glucocorticoid and mineralocorticoid deficiency. Mineralocorticoids are hormones produced in the adrenal cortex that control salt and water secretion from the kidney. The physiological functions of glucocorticoids, listed in *Table 7.3*, help to explain the side-effects of long-term treatment with oral glucocorticoids and the clinical features of Cushing's Syndrome, a condition caused by overproduction of endogenous glucocorticoids due to tumors of the adrenal cortex. The side effects of long term treatment with high dose glucocorticoids include cataracts, redistribution of fat, muscle wasting, hypertension, diabetes mellitus, skin thinning, easy bruising and loss of bone density.

The therapeutic potential of glucocorticoids in asthma as well as a number of other inflammatory conditions has long been recognized. Adrenal extracts were first used to treat asthmatics in 1900. The awareness that their beneficial effects were accompanied by less desirable results led to a number of modifications to the basic glucocorticoid structure in order to try and maximize the therapeutic effects and minimize the side-effects. A considerable breakthrough came in the early 1970s with the

Table 7.3: Physiological actions of glucocorticoids

1. Maintenance of blood glucose and liver glycogen levels
2. Maintenance of cardiovascular function, blood pressure and muscle work capacity
3. Excretion of water load
4. Permissive effect on lipolytic and gluconeogenic hormones
5. Protection against bodily stress

development of steroids that were topically active but had fewer systemic side-effects either because they were poorly absorbed through the gut or because they were rapidly metabolized in the liver. The structure of some of these molecules is illustrated in *Figure 7.2*. Given by aerosol they have been shown to be highly effective and relatively free of side-effects, the most troublesome of which is oral candidiasis. The standard aerosol delivery system is a pressurized canister that gives a fixed dose on actuation, the metered dose inhaler, although for many people it is difficult to co-ordinate actuation of the inhaler and inhalation. Further significant advances in management have been obtained with the development of inhalers which are easier to use, usually involving inhalation of powder rather than a spray. Even when used properly less than 10% of the drug is deposited in the airways, with most of it being swallowed. The amount reaching the airways can be doubled by using a spacer device.

Glucocorticoids exert their actions by passively diffusing into the cytoplasm and binding to a receptor protein called the glucocorticoid receptor.

The glucocorticoid receptor. Most cells, including all leukocytes, contain the glucocorticoid receptor (GR) in their cytoplasm. The potency of the various synthetic glucocorticoids correlates with their affinity for the GR. Binding of glucocorticoid to the GR results in activation of the receptor so that it moves into the nucleus, where it binds certain regions of DNA. The unactivated cytoplasmic form of the glucocorticoid receptor exists as a complex of proteins, which include two 90-kDa heat shock proteins (HSPs) and an approximately 96-kDa protein that contains the glucocorticoid- and DNA-binding regions (*Figure 7.3*). HSPs are a family of cytoplasmic regulatory proteins that control transport and organization of a number of proteins within the cell. The DNA-binding domain of the glucocorticoid receptor proper has a region of high cysteine content homologous to regions of proteins that regulate gene transcription (transcriptional factors) called 'zinc fingers'. Zinc fingers are thought to mediate protein binding to DNA. The human glucocorticoid receptor is related to a family of hormone receptors that includes the thyroid hormone receptor, the mineralocorticoid receptor and the estrogen receptor. These in turn are members of a gene superfamily that includes the receptor for retinoic acid. Interestingly, if the glucocorticoid-binding region of the GR is replaced by the estrogen-binding region of the estrogen receptor to make a chimeric receptor, estrogen can then activate a glucocorticoid-responsive gene.

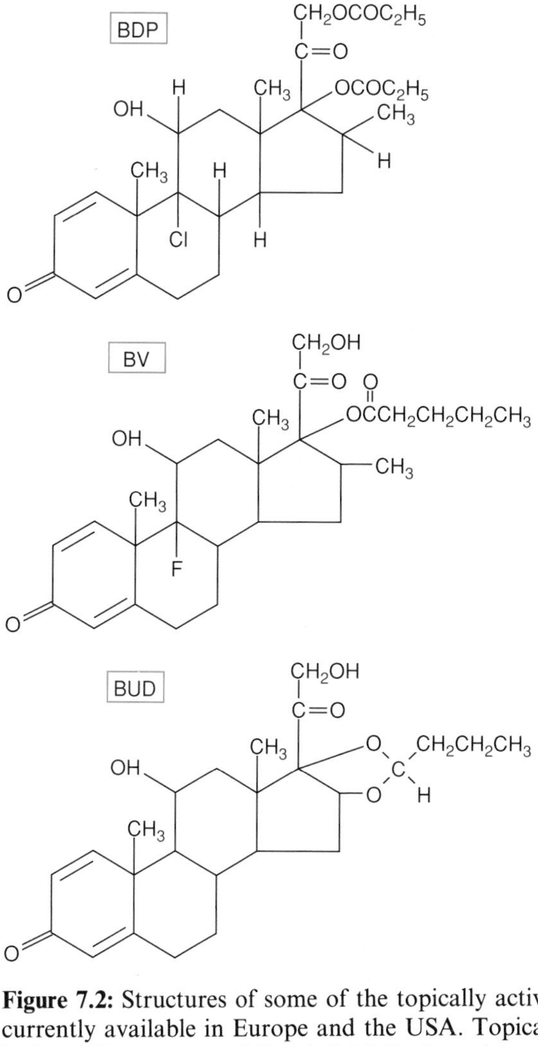

Figure 7.2: Structures of some of the topically active inhaled glucocorticoids currently available in Europe and the USA. Topical activity is conferred by the hydrophilic groups at C-7 and C-16. Beclomethasone (BDP) is chlorinated at C-9 and betamethasone (BV) has a fluoride atom. BUD = budesonide.

The current model of GR function suggests that binding of the glucocorticoid to the GR causes dissociation of the two HSPs, so changing the conformation of the GR complex, which migrates to the nucleus where it binds certain regions of DNA called glucocorticoid responsive elements (GREs) (*Figure 7.3*). This results in an increase or decrease in the rate of transcription of genes adjacent to the GREs as a result of interaction with enhancer and promoter regions. Some genes whose transcription is modified by glucocorticoids are listed in *Table 7.4*. GREs which result in increased transcription have a consensus sequence consisting of GGTACANNNTGTTCT (where N represents any nucleo-

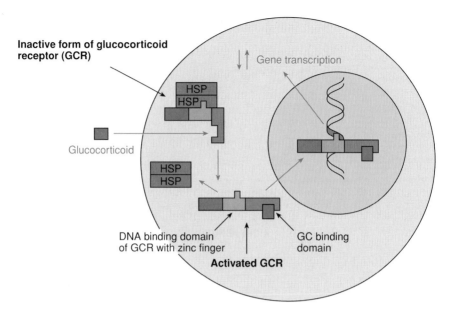

Figure 7.3: Simplified, schematic outline of the structure of the glucocorticoid receptor and its mechanism of action. Glucocorticoid passes into the cell and binds to the glucocorticoid-binding region of the receptor. This induces a conformational change in the receptor which results in it shedding its two associated heat shock proteins (HSPs), thereby exposing the zinc finger DNA-binding region of the receptor, which then moves into the nucleus where it binds to specific regions of DNA (glucocorticoid-responsive elements, GREs). Binding of the GR to GREs either represses or enhances transcription of the associated genes. Adapted from Munck *et al.* (1990) and Gustafsson *et al.* (1987).

tide). Inhibitory regions are more variable in their nucleotide sequence. Inhibitory effects of GC on protein synthesis can also occur at the post-translational level. One family of proteins that has been thought to be important in the anti-inflammatory actions of glucocorticoids is the lipocortins.

Lipocortin. Twenty years ago it was noted that glucocorticoids were able to inhibit synthesis of prostaglandins by inhibiting the activity of the enzyme phospholipase A_2, which releases arachidonic acid from glycero-phospholipids. It was subsequently determined that this effect was mediated by a protein called lipocortin 1 that is induced in a variety of glucocorticoid-treated cells. Lipocortin 1 is a 40 kDa calcium- and phospholipid-binding protein that is structurally related to a number of other calcium- and phospholipid-binding proteins of ill-defined function which are sometimes called annexins. In particular, these proteins share a 70-amino-acid repeating unit (repeated four times in lipocortin) in which the calcium- and phospholipid-binding sites are located. Crucial to lipocortin function is the 30-amino-acid N-terminal region, which is

Table 7.4: Products of glucocorticoid-responsive genes

Enhanced	Repressed
Lipocortin	IL-1*
β₂-Adrenoreceptor	TNF-α
Dihydrofolate reductase	GM-CSF
Metallothionein	IL-2
Growth hormone	IL-3
	IFN-γ
	IL-6
	IL-8

*As well as repressing gene transcription, glucocorticoids have effects at a post-transcriptional level, for example on stability of mRNA. With many cytokines, such as IL-1, effects on translation and protein processing are the more important pathways of repression of protein synthesis and secretion.

readily inactivated, an effect which can confound studies with the purified protein.

The mechanism by which lipocortin inhibits phospholipase A_2 is unclear. Its effects may be due in part to binding and sequestration of the phospholipid substrate. The role of lipocortin in mediating the anti-inflammatory properties of glucocorticoids in asthma is also still uncertain. Purified recombinant lipocortin can inhibit eicosanoid release from some, though not all, cell systems (for example, peritoneal macrophages stimulated with opsonized zymosan) as well as organ cultures such as the guinea pig lung. It is also able to inhibit some animal models of inflammation in which eicosanoids are important and are inhibited by glucocorticoids, such as the inflammatory response induced in the rat paw by an irritant called carrageenin. However, in other glucocorticoid-responsive systems it is ineffective. Increased amounts of lipocortin have not been detected in asthmatics, although there is some evidence that administration of glucocorticoids increases the amounts of lipocortin in the human lung. The results of treating inflammatory disease with purified lipocortin are awaited with interest.

Glucocorticoids and asthma. Glucocorticoids are very effective in treating asthma, and it is assumed that they exert their effect through suppressing airways inflammation. They are one of the few anti-asthma drugs that reduce bronchial hyperresponsiveness, although this can take several weeks for maximum effect. Which of the many anti-inflammatory effects of glucocorticoids are responsible for their success in asthma is still unclear. Definition of the pathways by which glucocorticoids work in asthma would give further clues to the pathogenesis of the disease as well as promoting the development of drugs which block that pathway without the unwelcome side-effects. The major actions of glucocorticoids of likely importance in asthma are listed in *Table 7.5*.

Table 7.5: Actions of glucocorticoids of importance in asthma

Cell type	Effect
Airways mast cells	No effects on IgE-mediated mast cell degranulation but several weeks' treatment with topical glucocorticoids reduces the numbers of airways mast cells
Basophils	Reduced numbers of circulating basophils and inhibition of basophil migration into nasal mucosa after allergen challenge
Eosinophils	Reduced numbers in peripheral blood and airways and reduced amounts of eosinophil granule proteins in BAL fluid from asthmatics
	Inhibition of cytokine-induced survival in *in vitro* culture
	Inhibition of cytokine-induced receptor expression
	Minimal effect on eosinophil degranulation
T lymphocytes	Marked inhibition of cytokine generation and proliferation
Monocytes/macrophages	Marked inhibition of generation of inflammatory mediators
Neutrophils	Generally fairly minimal effects. Treatment with oral glucocorticoids results in modest neutrophilia
Endothelium	Reduced microvascular leakage
Other effects	Reduction in bronchial hyperresponsiveness
	Increased responsiveness of bronchial smooth muscle to β_2-agonists

Oral prednisolone causes a marked fall in the number of circulating eosinophils (eosinopenia), and both inhaled and oral glucocorticoids reduce the number and activation status of eosinophils in the airways of asthmatics after allergen challenge and in steady-state disease. This is of obvious relevance to asthma, and indeed has been used as evidence for the importance of eosinophils in the disease. Although glucocorticoids do have direct effects on eosinophils at physiological doses (i.e. 10^{-6} to 10^{-7} M, which are concentrations likely to be found in the tissues), such as inhibition of membrane receptor expression and inhibition of cytokine-induced survival, the cells which appear most sensitive to the actions of glucocorticoids are monocytes and T lymphocytes. Glucocorticoids inhibit T-cell proliferation and cytokine release and inhibit the generation of a number of cytokines from monocytes and macrophages. An important pathway of glucocorticoid action is therefore likely to be inhibition of eosinophil migration into the lungs by inhibiting Th2-cell activation (see *Figure 7.3*). In support of this idea it has been shown that oral glucocorticoids result in decreased expression of mRNA for IL-4 and IL-5 in bronchoalveolar lavage cells from asthmatics, while a small increase in the number of T cells expressing gamma-interferon (IFN-γ) is observed. These effects are accompanied by a fall in the number of airway eosinophils and a corresponding improvement in lung function and bronchial hyperresponsiveness. This suggests the intriguing possibility that Th2 cells in asthmatic airways are more responsive to the inhibitory effects of glucocorticoids than Th1 cells.

Glucocorticoid resistance. As discussed in Chapter 1, some otherwise typical asthmatics do not appear to respond to glucocorticoids either symptomatically or in terms of lung function. While there is a range of response to glucocorticoids, a small number of asthmatics, in the region of 1%, do seem qualitatively different in that they fail to respond at all. As a group they tend to be older and their disease more severe. They absorb and metabolize glucocorticoids normally.

Glucocorticoid resistance is associated with a defect in the response of the asthmatic's peripheral blood T cells and monocytes to glucocorticoids *in vitro*, with glucocorticoids failing to inhibit lectin-induced proliferation and cytokine release from T cells and spontaneous production of a neutrophil-activating factor from monocytes. These patients have no clinical evidence of glucocorticoid deficiency or high cortisol and ACTH levels, as seen in a rare condition called familial glucocorticoid resistance, which is due to a single amino acid substitution in the hormone-binding region of the receptor. However, there is evidence of a global defect as patients are also found to be resistant to the skin blanching properties of glucocorticoids. When applied to the skin for a prolonged period (about 18 h) glucocorticoids cause vasoconstriction which can be readily detected as skin blanching. The effect is thought to be GR mediated and is used to test the relative potency of glucocorticoids. This suggests that the defect in glucocorticoid resistance lies in the GR. The affinity of binding of glucocorticoids to the GR appears to be lower in this group of patients, but the difference is small and its clinical importance is unclear. Recent evidence suggests that the defect may lie in the DNA-binding region of the receptor.

Although glucocorticoid resistance is uncommon, its recognition is clinically important in avoiding inappropriate use of glucocorticoids. In addition, unraveling the molecular basis of glucocorticoid resistance may help to define more precisely the mechanism of action of these powerful drugs in asthma.

7.2.2 Disodium cromoglycate (DSCG) and nedocromil

DSCG was developed as a result of investigations into the bronchodilator properties of Khellin, an isolate from the seeds of a Mediterranean herb, *Ammi visnagi*, which was known for its smooth muscle relaxant properties. DSCG is a bis-chromone (*Figure 7.4*). During early development, DSCG was found to inhibit both the early and the late response to allergen challenge and was later found to be effective in the treatment of chronic asthma.

DSCG is a relatively inert compound with little biological activity, which means that it has very few side-effects. One property of obvious relevance is its ability to inhibit mast cell degranulation induced either by cross-linking IgE or by secretagogues such as calcium ionophore, and it had been assumed that this was the reason why it is effective in the treatment of asthma. In support of this theory is the observation that it

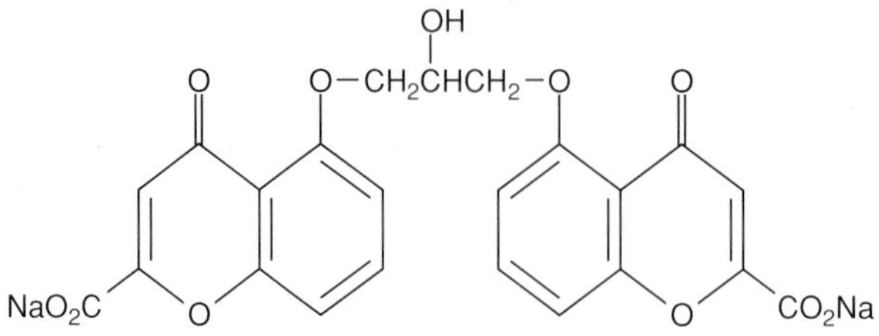

Figure 7.4: Structure of disodium cromoglycate.

can inhibit bronchoconstriction induced by exercise, cold air challenge and hyperventilation, which is thought to be mediated by mast cell degranulation. However, a number of drugs that are more potent 'mast cell stabilizers' have been developed which are ineffective in treating asthma. β_2-Agonists, which are more potent mast cell stabilizers than DSCG, have little anti-inflammatory activity in that they have no effect on the leukocyte infiltration into the lung in asthma and they do not improve bronchial hyperresponsiveness.

DSCG has subsequently been found to have a number of other actions, including inhibition of eosinophil and neutrophil priming by mediators such as PAF and inhibition of neural reflexes within the lung. The precise mechanism of action of DSCG in asthma is therefore unclear. DSCG is genuinely anti-inflammatory in that it reduces the number of eosinophils in the airways of asthmatics and prevents the development of bronchial hyperresponsiveness during the pollen season in seasonal asthmatics. Although it is undoubtedly beneficial in the treatment of asthma, especially in the management of milder, young asthmatics, and free of side-effects, DSCG is not a particularly active drug and appears to be completely ineffective in many adult patients. The effectiveness and safety of inhaled steroids has rather overshadowed its role in treating asthma. Many drug companies have devoted considerable resources to producing a follow-up drug to DSCG which would have greater effectiveness. This has been largely unsuccessful, with only nedocromil sodium being fully developed and marketed. Although structurally different to DSCG, it appears to have a very similar profile of activity both *in vitro* and *in vivo* in asthma.

7.3 Current therapies for asthma: bronchodilators

7.3.1 β_2-Agonists

The adrenergic system consists of the sympathetic nervous system, catecholamines and the α- and β-adrenergic membrane receptors. Catecholamines include norepinephrine (noradrenaline), which is released from the sympathetic nerve endings, and epinephrine (adrenaline), which comes from the adrenal medulla. α-Receptor stimulation causes smooth muscle constriction and β-receptor stimulation causes relaxation. There are at least two types of β-receptors, β_1 and β_2. In humans β_1-receptors are found in the heart, whereas bronchial smooth muscle, although not receiving any sympathetic nerve fibers, is rich in β_2-receptors. Norepinephrine and epinephrine are non-selective in their actions so that bronchodilation is accompanied by cardiac side-effects, including increased heart rate and force of contraction. Similarly, non-selective β-antagonists (β-blockers) cause bronchoconstriction. Interestingly β-blocker-induced bronchoconstriction is seen only in asthmatics, although hitherto unrecognized asthma may be revealed in a mild sufferer. It is well recognized that this can occur even with β-blockers in eye drops for glaucoma. The observation that β-blockers affect only asthmatics suggests that persistent β_2-receptor stimulation is required to prevent smooth muscle contraction in asthma. Although bronchodilation is less prominent with the more selective β_1-blockers, these drugs are best avoided in any asthmatic. The catecholamines are very short-acting, being rapidly reabsorbed into the nerve axon, where they are stored or metabolized by monoamine oxidase. Alternatively, they are methylated by catechol-*O*-methyltransferase.

β_2-Receptors. The β_2-adrenergic receptor is a member of the gene family of seven-transmembrane G protein-linked receptors. Stimulation results in G-protein activation leading to activation of adenylate cyclase and increased levels of cyclic AMP (see Chapter 3). As well as being expressed on bronchial smooth muscle, β_2-receptors are expressed on the airways epithelium, including Clara cells, and on the submucosal mucus glands. β_2-agonists cause mucus hypersecretion *in vitro*, although this does not appear to be a prominent effect *in vivo*.

Mast cells and leukocytes also express β_2-receptors, and β_2-agonists are potent inhibitors of mast cell degranulation. Theoretically, therefore, they could be thought of as having anti-inflammatory activity. However, fiber-optic studies have not provided any evidence of an anti-inflammatory effect of this class of drugs *in vivo*, and they may even increase bronchial hyperresponsiveness.

An important feature of β_2-receptor function is desensitization. Thus, cells exposed to β_2-agonists become unresponsive to further challenge. The duration of unresponsiveness depends on the concentration and duration of the initial stimulus. There are two phases. Acute unresponsiveness occurs after about 60 min exposure to 0.01 μM isoprenaline as a result of phosphorylation of the receptor, which beomes uncoupled from adenylate cyclase. This abates relatively quickly, unlike a more chronic unresponsiveness seen at higher concentrations of β_2-agonist, which is due to decreased expression of the receptor. The extent to which this occurs *in vivo* and is relevant to β_2-agonist treatment in asthma is uncertain. Asthmatics appear to be less prone to β_2-agonist tachyphylaxis than non-asthmatics. There is also no evidence that expression of the β_2-receptor is reduced in airways smooth muscle in asthma, although airways smooth muscle in patients who have died from asthma appears relatively unresponsive to β_2-agonists.

Glucocorticoids restore β_2-receptor function after desensitization within a few hours of administration, and this is one rationale for giving glucocorticoids as quickly as possible in acute severe asthma. Desensitization is of potential relevance to the development of long-acting β_2-agonists which bind to the receptor for many hours.

Synthetic β_2-agonists. The main aim of drug development in the field of β_2-agonists has been more specific and longer acting drugs than the naturally occurring catecholamines. A number of very successful compounds have been developed with varying potencies lasting between 4 and 6 h. These are active at low doses by an inhaled route and as such have few side-effects. They are one of the mainstays of asthma therapy. These drugs are also effective orally although they then have more side-effects, particularly tremor and tachycardia, the latter caused by β_1-agonist activity. The structures of some of these compounds are shown in *Figure 7.5*. More recently, compounds that are active for more than 12 h have been developed, and these have been shown to be well tolerated and effective, particularly in the treatment of nocturnal symptoms.

In recent years the safety of β_2-agonists has been questioned. An epidemic of asthma deaths in the UK was associated with an increase in

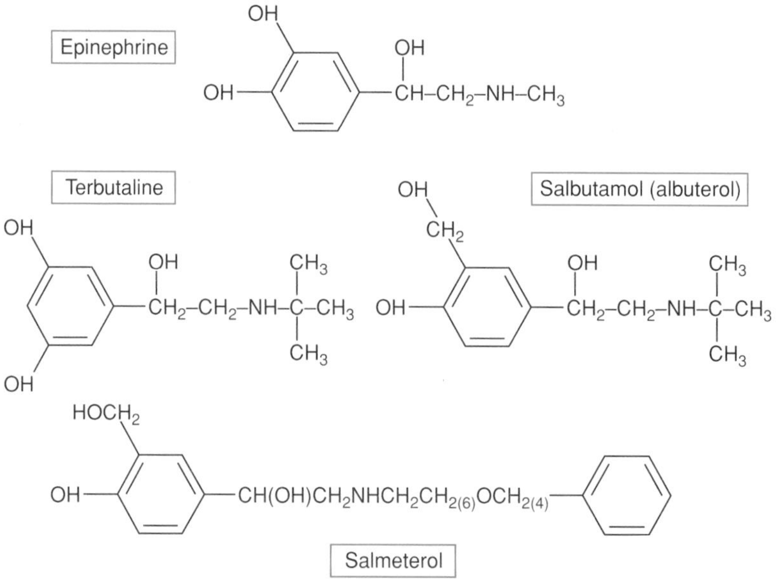

Figure 7.5: Comparison of the structures of epinephrine (adrenaline) with three of the β_2-agonists currently used in clinical practice. The long lipid tail of salmeterol confers its prolonged activity, possibly by anchoring the receptor and drug in the cell membrane.

the use of isoprenaline metered dose inhalers, and studies from New Zealand and Canada have provided evidence for a link between asthma deaths and the use of fenoterol, a potent and relatively non-selective and long-acting β_2-agonist. These associations could just as well be interpreted as showing that severe asthmatics, at risk of dying, tend to rely more on their β_2-agonists, and case studies have suggested that a contributory cause in many asthma deaths is lack of recognition of the severity of an attack and undertreatment with glucocorticoids. However, the regular use of fenoterol was shown in one study to result in poorer control of asthma than intermittent use. These studies are far from conclusive. Nonetheless, there have been case reports of attacks of acute severe asthma for the first time in people taking salmeterol, a new long-acting inhaled β_2-agonist. A large community-based study comparing salmeterol with salbutamol found no significant difference in asthma deaths or attacks of acute severe asthma between the two groups. More studies to clarify some of these issues are clearly needed.

7.3.2 Theophylline

Theophylline is a naturally occurring alkaloid deriving its name from the Greek for 'divine leaf' in tribute to the leaves of the tea plant. It is a dimethylxanthine and is closely related to theobromine, which is found in cocoa seeds, and caffeine (*Figure 7.6*). The medicinal effects of this group of drugs were first noted in 1859, when it was reported that strong black coffee was one of the best treatments for attacks of asthma. Theophylline had been chemically identified by the late nineteenth century, but it was not routinely used in the treatment of asthma until the late 1930s. It has been widely used ever since for its bronchodilator properties in both chronic asthma, when it is given by the oral or rectal route, and acute severe asthma, when it is administered intravenously.

Theophylline salts have been used to improve solubility, but only aminophylline (ethylenediamine + theophylline) and choline theophyllinate (choline + theophylline) are used clinically to any extent. These dissociate *in vivo* into free theophylline and the cation.

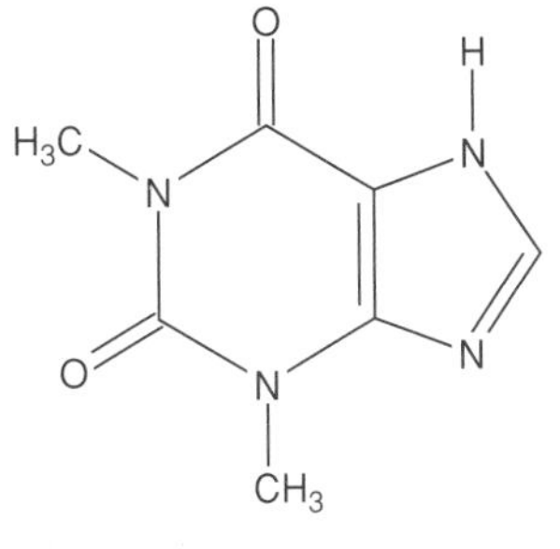

Figure 7.6: Structure of theophylline.

Theophylline is an effective bronchodilator, but its use has been limited by its narrow therapeutic window. It appears to exert its therapeutic effect only between 5 and 20 $\mu g\ ml^{-1}$; above 20 $\mu g\ ml^{-1}$ its toxic effects, which include potentially fatal cardiac arrhythmias and epileptogenic fits, become increasingly likely, particularly with intravenous therapy. The main side-effect limiting oral use is gastric intolerance. In addition, the evidence for a benefit of theophyllines over and above effectively delivered topical β_2-agonists is not convincing. For this reason theophyllines have fallen out of favor to some degree, although they are still widely used in severe attacks of asthma and are one of the most commonly prescribed oral anti-asthma medications worldwide.

Mechanism of action. Theophyllines are relatively weak and non-selective inhibitors of a family of enzymes called cyclic nucleotide phosphodiesterases (CN-PDEs). These enzymes hydrolyze cyclic AMP (cAMP) and cyclic GMP (cGMP) to their non-cyclic monophosphates, so PDE inhibitors increase levels of cyclic nucleotides, leading to bronchodilation (*Figure 7.7*). However, theophyllines appear to cause smooth muscle relaxation at 10- to 20-fold lower concentrations than that required for PDE inhibition. In addition, more potent PDE inhibitors have no bronchodilatory activity. Some of these discrepancies may be explained by the different properties of PDE isoenzymes, discussed below.

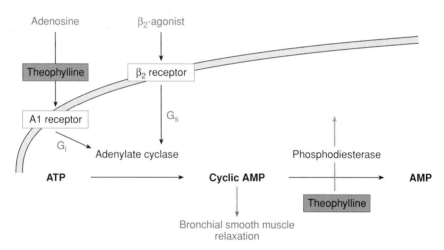

Figure 7.7: Mechanism of action of theophylline. Increased levels of the cyclic nucleotides cAMP and cGMP in the cytoplasm result in relaxation of bronchial smooth muscle. cAMP is generated from ATP by the action of adenylate cyclase activated by stimulatory G proteins associated with a number of membrane receptors including the β_2-agonist receptor. Other receptors, such as one of the adenosine receptors, are associated with inhibitory G proteins (G_i), which lead to inhibition of adenylate cyclase, decreased levels of cAMP and bronchoconstriction. Theophylline inhibits phosphodiesterase (which metabolizes cyclic nucleotides) and also antagonizes adenosine binding to its receptor.

Theophylline also antagonizes adenosine by competitively binding to adenosine receptors. Adenosine is a naturally occurring purine nucleoside that is released in the airways after allergen challenge. It has two receptors: A1, which is linked to an inhibitory G protein that reduces levels of adenylate cyclase; and A2, which is associated with a stimulatory G protein that increases levels of adenylate cyclase. Binding to both receptors is antagonized by theophylline. The A1 receptor is responsible for mediating smooth muscle contraction. Inhaled adenosine causes bronchoconstriction in asthmatics but not normal subjects, and theophylline prevents this at concentrations lower than that required to cause bronchodilation. However, anprofylline is a more potent bronchodilator than theophylline in man and has no adenosine antagonistic properties. Elevation of cAMP prevents degranulation of mast cells and mediator release from granulocytes and macrophages, suggesting that theophylline could have anti-inflammatory activity. However, there is no *in vivo* evidence for an anti-inflammatory effect of theophylline, and theophylline, unlike glucocorticoids, fails to reduce airways hyperresponsiveness after several weeks' treatment.

7.3.3 Anti-cholinergics

The majority of the autonomic nerves in the lung are cholinergic, derived from the vagal nerve. Branches of the vagal nerve run along the bronchi, predominantly in the larger airways, to peribronchial ganglia, from which they send out short post-ganglionic fibers to smooth muscle cells and mucus glands. Acetylcholine released from the stimulated nerve endings binds to muscarinic receptors in the membrane of the smooth muscle, which leads to bronchoconstriction.

Muscarinic receptors are members of the family of seven-transmembrane domain G protein-linked receptors. There are a number of subtypes, of which M1, M2 and M3 have been well characterized. M2 receptors are linked to adenylate cyclase through an inhibitory G protein (G_i), which results in decreased levels of cyclic nucleotides, whereas M3 uses phosphatidylinositol as second messengers (see Chapter 3). Muscarinic receptors appear to be exclusively of the M3 subtype in human bronchial smooth muscle.

Anti-cholinergic drugs have been used for centuries in the treatment of asthma. Four thousand years ago in India a herbal remedy derived from the plant *Nardostachys jatamansi*, which contains an anti-cholinergic alkaloid, was inhaled for the treatment of respiratory disease. In the nineteenth century belladonna leaves (which contain the anti-cholinergic atropine), extracts of the Indian herb *Datura stramonium* and hyoscyamine were commonly used to treat asthma. Stramonium was the preferred drug until it was supplanted by inhaled epinephrine in the 1930s. Use of anti-cholinergics was limited because of side-effects of dry mouth, flushing, lightheadedness and blurred vision.

The quaternary derivatives of atropine, ipratropium bromide and oxitropium bromide, are more specific bronchodilators and have found a place in the management of asthma (*Figure 7.8*). They are generally less effective bronchodilators than β_2-agonists and have a more delayed onset of action although their effect is more prolonged.

Response to anti-cholinergics is rather unpredictable, with some patients showing very little response and others marked bronchodilation. The reason for this is not clear. Anti-cholinergics are often more effective bronchodilators than β_2-agonists in patients with smoking-related airflow obstruction. Anti-cholinergics are generally well tolerated with few systemic side-effects as they are poorly absorbed, although there is a risk of precipitating urinary retention and glaucoma at high doses in older patients. The currently available anti-cholinergics are non-specific blockers of muscarinic receptors. It remains to be seen whether selective M3 antagonists will have an improved profile of activity.

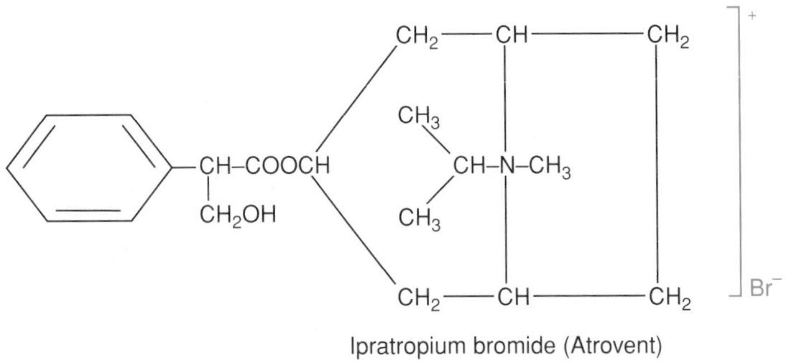

Ipratropium bromide (Atrovent)

Figure 7.8: Structure of the anti-cholinergic, ipratropium bromide.

7.4 New treatments for asthma

7.4.1 Introduction

The treatments described above are very effective at both relieving and preventing airflow obstruction and have a generally good side-effect profile. Treatment failures are more often to do with poor compliance and inappropriate inhaler devices than inability of the drugs to control the disease. It is therefore debatable whether new drugs for the treatment of asthma are needed. However, the approximately 1% of asthmatics, many of whom are children, who remain difficult to control on current treatment make up a significant number of patients. There is still considerable morbidity and a certain mortality to the disease which will be difficult to eradicate with the present therapeutic armamentarium, even with universally optimum management. There are still many patients who suffer major long-term side-effects from oral corticosteroids.

The advances in our understanding of the nature of the inflammatory response that characterizes asthma has opened the way for a range of new, more specifically targeted, anti-inflammatory drugs. These include inhibitors of T-lymphocyte function such as cyclosporine (CsA), antimetabolites which inhibit all leukocytes, such as methotrexate, anti-adhesion molecules, and anti-mediator drugs such as IL-5 antagonists. However, none of these is likely to offer a cure. We are still some distance from understanding the fundamental defects that cause asthma. Perhaps the most promising area in this regard is the work being undertaken to define the exact nature of the T-cell response to allergen. Coupled with our understanding of the mechanism of T-cell activation, it offers the possibility of switching off or diverting this response, possibly by immunization with modified allergens that render the T cell anergic to natural stimuli.

7.4.2 Immunosuppressants

Cyclosporine, rapamycin and FK-506. Cyclosporine was originally isolated from cultures of the fungus *Tolypocladium inflatum* and attracted widespread interest when it was found to have marked immunosuppressive activity without suppressing the bone marrow. This was a major breakthrough in preventing rejection of transplanted organs and it has since been found to be effective in a range of chronic inflammatory conditions, including psoriasis, Crohn's disease, Behçet's disease and atopic dermatitis. CsA has a number of side-effects, including hypertrichosis, hepatotoxicity and renal impairment, which can be irreversible.

FK-506 was isolated from the fermentation broth of *Streptomyces tsukubaensis*, an organism found in the soil in Japan. Like rapamycin, it is a macrolide that is structurally unrelated to CsA. It has a similar profile of activity to CsA *in vivo*, but appears to be more potent.

Rapamycin was discovered as an antifungal agent in the fermentation broth of *Streptomyces hygroscopicus*, originally isolated from a soil sample from Easter Island (Rapa Nui). It was first developed as an antibiotic, although its immunosuppressive properties were soon recognized. However, it was not used as an immunosuppressant until recently when structural similarities between FK-506 and rapamycin were noted.

CsA and FK-506 are highly effective at inhibiting T-cell proliferation induced by a number of signals, including signaling through the T-cell antigen receptor. They appear to work by inhibiting transcription of the genes for several cytokines, including IL-2, IL-3 and IL-4. IL-2 production by the T cell is essential for proliferation to occur, and the effects of these drugs can be overcome to some extent by adding exogenous IL-2. IL-2 synthesis occurs early in T-cell proliferation, and consistent with this CsA and FK-506 are only effective if given prior to, or very shortly after, T-cell stimulation. In contrast, rapamycin does not affect cytokine generation by T cells but appears to act at a later point in the cell cycle.

The molecular basis of the action of these drugs is providing interesting insights on mechanisms of leukocyte activation. They bind to a family of abundant cellular proteins called immunophilins, which have wide tissue distribution and are characterized by having proline isomerase activity (PPIase) and are thought to be important in protein folding. They have been highly conserved throughout evolution, with one member in *Drosophila* being important for rhodopsin synthesis. The prototype of the immunophilin family is an 18-kDa molecule that binds CsA, called cyclophilin. Rapamycin and FK-506 bind a related molecule called FK-binding protein (FKBP). Inhibition of immunophilin PPIase activity does not appear to be the basis for the action of CsA, FK-506 and rapamycin. Analogs of cyclosporine have been identified that are effective at inhibiting the PPIase activity of cyclophilin but have little immunosuppressive activity. In contrast, another analog is immunosuppressive but binds weakly to cyclophilin. In addition, although FK-506 and rapamycin share the same binding protein, they have a different mechanism of immunosuppression. It appears that the CsA–cyclophilin and FK-506–FKBP complexes inhibit the actions of a calcium/calmodulin-dependent protein phosphatase (an enzyme that dephosphorylates proteins) called calcineurin (also called PP2B). Calcineurin is involved in transducing the initial signal from the T-cell antigen receptor, which results in IL-2 expression and transition of the cell from the resting G_0 phase to the G_1 phase of the cell cycle. It seems likely that the rapamycin–FKBP complex inhibits the function of a related phosphatase that mediates signal transduction following IL-2 (or other growth factors) binding to its receptor, which is responsible for the cell moving from G_1 to the next, S, phase of the cell cycle (*Figure 7.9*).

Few studies have been performed with these drugs in asthma. In a well-designed and carefully executed, double-blind, placebo-controlled study, CsA at a relatively low dose was found to improve lung function in a group of severely affected, steroid-dependent asthmatics, a remarkable achievement in view of the resistance of this group of patients to treatment. This was seen as supporting the hypothesis that T lymphocytes are central to asthma pathogenesis, although CsA is also able to inhibit the function of most leukocytes as well as preventing mast cell degranulation and cytokine production. Treatment with CsA may have a place in the management of the severe steroid-dependent asthmatic, but more widespread use of this class of drugs will have to await compounds with better side-effect profiles.

Methotrexate. Methotrexate is a folate antagonist that binds with high affinity to dihydrofolate reductase, so inhibiting the synthesis of nucleic acids, amino acids and essential fatty acids. It is structurally very similar to folate. Originally used in oncology as an anti-neoplastic drug because of its ability to inhibit cell division, it was then found at lower doses to be an effective anti-inflammatory agent for the treatment of psoriasis and

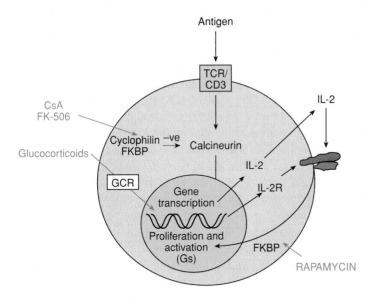

Figure 7.9: Mechanism of action of the immunosuppressive drugs cyclosporine A, FK-506 and rapamycin. These drugs bind to the immunophilins cyclophilin and FKBP, and the drug–immunophilin complex inhibits the signal transduction events resulting from antigen binding to the T-cell antigen receptor. CsA and FK-506 inhibit calcineurin, a calcium-dependent phosphatase that mediates the initial signal which results in cytokine synthesis and the cell moving from the G_0 to the G_1 phase. The rapamycin–FKBP complex inhibits a putative calcineurin-like phosphatase, so preventing the signal transduction resulting from IL-2 and other growth factors binding to their receptors, which moves the cell from the G_1 to the G_s cell division phase. The site of action of these drugs is therefore distinct from that of glucocorticoids, which have a more direct effect on gene transcription.

rheumatoid arthritis. Using a low-dose regimen with avoidance of alcohol and careful monitoring, side-effects, which include bone marrow suppression, cirrhosis and hepatic and pulmonary fibrosis, are unusual. Double-blind placebo-controlled studies have demonstrated that methotrexate is effective as a steroid-sparing agent in severe oral glucocorticoid-dependent asthmatics. Mean reductions in oral glucocorticoid usage of the order of 50% have been achieved, with a number of patients being able to stop oral glucocorticoids altogether. However, the required dose of glucocorticoids once again increases when the methotrexate treatment is stopped. The mechanism of action of the anti-inflammatory effects of low-dose methotrexate is not entirely clear. One effect may be through inhibition of leukocyte migration into the airways as it effectively inhibits leukocyte chemotaxis *in vitro*. Again, although methotrexate may have a place in the treatment of the very severe asthmatic, it has a number of major side-effects and its efficacy, although clearly demonstrated, is not dramatic.

7.4.3 Bronchodilators

Phosphodiesterase inhibitors. Phosphodiesterases (PDEs) are a family of enzymes that metabolize and inactivate the second messengers cAMP and cGMP. Five classes of PDEs have been defined biochemically (*Table 7.6*). PDE inhibitors increase cAMP levels, leading to a variety of effects, from relaxation of bronchial smooth muscle to inhibition of leukocyte activation and mediator release. The principal actions of theophylline are likely to be due to its non-selective PDE inhibitory activity. It is hoped that selective and potent PDE inhibitors will be more effective than theophylline and not share its side-effects.

The major bronchodilating PDEs in bronchial smooth muscle are types III and IV, whereas the principal leukocyte PDE is type IV. In bronchial smooth muscle, type III PDE inhibition is more closely correlated with bronchodilation. Like theophylline and β_2-agonists, selective PDE inhibitors are functional bronchodilators in that they cause bronchial smooth muscle relaxation whatever the spasmogen. PDE inhibitors, particularly type IV-selective drugs such as rolipram, are able to inhibit leukocyte function. For example, rolipram inhibits the respiratory burst and oxygen radical production by eosinophils stimulated with opsonized zymosan or LTB_4. This suggests that these drugs may have some anti-inflammatory activity as well as being bronchodilators. However, there is no *in vivo* evidence for this.

The effectiveness of selective PDE inhibitors in asthma awaits evaluation. As with theophyllines, one problem may be a high incidence of side-effects, with type III inhibitors causing problematic cardiovascular side-effects, including hypotension and tachycardia, and type IV inhibitors causing nausea and gastric upset.

Table 7.6: Selective PDE inhibitors

PDE family	Preferred substrate	Cell type	Inhibitor
I	Cyclic AMP		Vinopocetine
II	No preference		No inhibitors
III	Cyclic AMP	T lymphocyte	SKF 94120
		Bronchial smooth muscle	Imazodan
		Platelet	Others
		Basophil	
IV	Cyclic AMP	Eosinophil	Rolipram
		Neutrophil	Ro 20-1724
		T lymphocyte	
		Endothelial cell (bovine)	
		Bronchial smooth muscle	
		Monocyte	
		Mast cell (mouse)	
		Basophil	
V	Cyclic GMP	Platelet	Zaprinast
		Neutrophil	SKF 96231

Potassium channel openers (KCOs). A number of drugs that open potassium channels and as a result cause smooth muscle relaxation have been developed. Some of these relax airways smooth muscle, both suppressing the spontaneous tone of human bronchial smooth muscle and antagonizing the effect of exogenous spasmogens. There are more than 10 types of potassium channel. The potassium channels opened by the KCOs such as cromakalim, which relax airways smooth muscle, may be ATPase sensitive, whereas relaxation via β_2-agonists and theophylline involves a calcium-activated potassium channel.

The exact mechanism by which KCOs cause bronchodilation is unclear. They inhibit calcium flux into the cell by blocking voltage-operated calcium channels, but nifedipine and verapamil, which also do this, have little effect on isolated airways smooth muscle. Despite its *in vitro* properties, lemakalim, the active metabolite of cromakalim, has no bronchodilating properties when given orally although it has a modest effect in attenuating the diurnal variation in peak flow in nocturnal asthma, the dose being limited by headaches. Interestingly, cromakalim is more effective at inhibiting histamine-induced bronchoconstriction in hyperreactive guinea pigs than in normoreactive animals. The effectiveness of this group of drugs may be limited by their cardiovascular side-effects, including tachycardia and hypotension.

7.4.4 Mediator antagonists

Introduction. The potential involvement of several mediators in asthma suggests that antagonism of just one or two may have a limited therapeutic effect and that the search for a single effective antagonist may be somewhat fruitless. However, at the very least, clinical trials of effective and specific antagonists allow further evaluation of the role of a mediator in disease, and it remains possible that one mediator is dominant. For an antagonist to be informative and potentially useful it has to be highly effective (i.e. block most of the activity of the mediator), specific, safe and well tolerated at the concentration required for mediator antagonism. It has to reach the target organ in amounts sufficient to achieve an inhibitory concentration and be sufficiently long-lasting to achieve a measurable effect. Mediator antagonists can either interfere with synthesis of a mediator, block binding to its receptor or increase its metabolism. In practice, nearly all antagonists fit into the first two categories.

Having developed such a drug it then has to be tested for activity in disease. A popular model for the testing of anti-asthma drugs is allergen challenge to the lung in sensitized animals or humans. The airflow obstruction seen in both the early- and late-phase response to allergen challenge is likely to be caused principally by mast cell-derived mediators. The early phase is due to the rapid release of bronchospastic mediators such as histamine, the sulfidopeptide leukotrienes and PGD_2. Although the late phase is associated with an influx of T cells, monocytes and eosinophils, much of the airflow obstruction seen during the late-phase response is probably the result of airways edema caused by vasoactive mediators released from mast cells. As we have seen, there is good evidence that the mast cell is only part of the inflammatory process in chronic asthma and may not even have a major role. Models such as allergen or exercise challenge which emphasize the role of the mast cell may therefore give a misleading picture as to the efficacy of the drug in chronic asthma. Caution should therefore be applied in extrapolating results from allergen challenge studies, especially in animal models, to clinical asthma.

Two mediators that have gained prominence during the 1980s as being potentially important in asthma are PAF and the sulfidopeptide leukotrienes, LTC_4, D_4 and E_4. Antagonists of these molecules are now beginning to be used in clinical trials. In the 1990s the role of cytokines has become more pronounced, and in the next few years it is hoped that effective antagonists against molecules such as IL-3, IL-4 and IL-5 will become available. However, at present, information on the potential usefulness of cytokine antagonists is limited to blocking monoclonal antibodies in animal models.

PAF antagonists. Trials with effective PAF antagonists have so far proved disappointing. Three synthetic PAF antagonists that block binding of PAF to its receptor, WEB-2086, UK-74,505 and MK-287, failed to inhibit either the early- or late-phase response to allergen in atopic individuals despite blocking PAF-induced platelet aggregation and bronchoconstriction. As there is little evidence that PAF is released by human lung mast cells after allergen challenge it could be argued that this is not altogether surprising. The acid test is whether PAF antagonists have any effect in clinical asthma, but information on this is limited. Ginkgolides are complex organic molecules, derived from the Ginkgo biloba tree, that have been used as traditional remedies for cough and wheeze. They are relatively weak PAF antagonists. There have been anecdotal reports that the compound BN52063, a mixture of ginkgolides, is effective in treating asthma, but these have never been well documented. However, WEB-2086 appeared to have no steroid-sparing activity over a 3-week period in asthmatics requiring inhaled steroids. Information on PAF antagonists is therefore still scanty, but the omens are not promising.

Leukotriene antagonists. Preliminary studies with leukotriene antagonists have been much more promising. Leukotriene D_4 receptor antagonists inhibit both the early and late response to allergen challenge in atopic individuals as well as exercise challenge. Both a 5-lipoxygenase inhibitor, Zileuton, and two LTD_4 receptor blockers, MK-571 and ICI 204,219, were able to improve lung function (7.5% increase in FEV_1 with oral ICI 204,219 and a 20% increase in FEV_1 following intravenous MK-571) in chronic asthmatics. Encouragingly, the effect was greater than that achieved with β_2-agonists. Preliminary reports of leukotriene antagonists in clinical asthma are also encouraging (*Table 7.7*).

Cytokine antagonists. Awareness of the central role of cytokines in inflammation in general and asthma in particular has raised the possibility that cytokine antagonists might be effective in the treatment of asthma. Unlike granule-stored mediators or newly synthesized membrane-derived mediators, cytokines are usually generated by *de novo* protein synthesis. Antagonists can therefore be designed to inhibit DNA transcription or protein synthesis as well as block receptors.

One rather futuristic-sounding approach to inhibition of protein synthesis is antisense drugs. These are oligonucleotides (short sections of single-stranded DNA, usually less than 50 nucleotides, which can be readily synthesized to order) which are designed to be identical to a section of the reverse (antisense) strand of the gene in question and therefore complementary to a section of the mRNA strand. The oligonucleotide binds specifically to the mRNA derived from the gene of interest and blocks translation of the mRNA into protein. Antisense technology is effective in the test tube and trials are beginning for the

Table 7.7: Leukotriene antagonists

| Antagonist | (Type % shift in dose response to LTD$_4$) | EIA | Allergen challenge | | Clinical asthma |
			Early	Late	
MK-571	LTD$_4$ receptor antagonist (30–40)	Inhibits	Inhibits	Inhibits (50%)	Single dose bronchodilates Improvement in lung function and symptom scores
ICI 204,219	LTD$_4$ receptor antagonist (100)	Inhibits	Inhibits	Inhibits (50%)	Single dose bronchodilates Improvement in lung function and symptom scores
RG12525	LTD$_4$ receptor antagonist	NR	NR	NR	Improvement in lung function and symptom scores
SKF-104,353	LTD$_4$ receptor antagonist (3–4)	Inhibits	Inhibits	Inhibits	NR
LY-171,883	LTD$_4$ receptor antagonist (3–4)	NR	Inhibits (weakly)		Small improvement in lung function
Zileuton	Lipoxygenase antagonist	NR	NR	NR	Moderately effective
MK-886	FLAP antagonist	NR	Inhibits	Inhibits	NR

FLAP, 5-lipoxygenase-activating protein; NR, not reported.

treatment of malignant conditions. One problem is access of the oligonucleotide to the cells producing the cytokine, but it is not too far-fetched to imagine a form of inhaled oligonucleotide, possibly carried in liposomes, being used for the treatment of asthma in the not too distant future.

In any case, the principal cytokines and their receptors have been fully characterized and the arrival of effective antagonists is eagerly awaited. However, to date no cytokine antagonists have reached the stage of clinical trials in asthma, and the only evidence for their potential effectiveness comes from the use of monoclonal antibodies in animal models. Monoclonal antibodies (mAbs) are antibodies raised in animals, usually mice, which have a single antigenic specificity. Any one mAb will recognize a single epitope of a single antigen. They are therefore highly specific tools for both research and therapeutics. If the mAb recognizes an epitope at or near a region important for the function of the molecule it will block that function (blocking antibodies). The problem with mouse-derived mAbs is that the antibody is a foreign antigen which could potentially provoke an immune response, limiting its effectiveness and possibly provoking problems greater than the disease being treated. This is less important if only short courses of treatment on a one-off basis are required, but could be a major problem for the treatment of a chronic inflammatory disease such as asthma. In fact, mouse mAbs directed against T lymphocytes are currently being used for renal transplant rejection, and anti-endotoxin mAbs are available for the treatment of Gram-negative septicemia. One way around the problem of sensitization is to engineer the antibody so that most of it is identical to human immunoglobulin and therefore non-antigenic, with only the antigen recognition part being derived from the mouse. Whether such antibodies will become part of routine clinical treatment remains to be seen.

A number of cytokines have been implicated in asthma, including IL-3, GM-CSF, TNF-α and chemokine cytokines such as RANTES and IL-8. However, the two that have received the most attention are the Th2-associated cytokines IL-4 and IL-5. IL-4 promotes IgE synthesis, Th2-lymphocyte activation and possibly eosinophil localization in tissues. IL-5 is the major cytokine involved in eosinophil production and also selectively stimulates the function of mature eosinophils.

mAbs against IL-5 abolish the eosinophil response to helminthic infection in mice, suggesting that IL-5 antagonists may be effective in preventing the production of eosinophils in the bone marrow. Whether this would have any immunosuppressive effects is uncertain, but individuals who seem to completely lack eosinophils and are perfectly healthy have been reported. mAbs given after allergen challenge in the guinea pig reduce the eosinophil influx into the lungs, which is evidence for a direct role for IL-5 in mediating eosinophil tissue accumulation in the airways. However, there are significant functional differences between guinea pig and human eosinophils, so that the guinea pig model is in many ways not ideal. Nonetheless, it seems likely that an effective IL-5 antagonist would greatly reduce if not abolish the eosinophilia of asthma, which at the very least should determine whether this cell is indeed important in the disease.

Anti-IL-4 mAbs inhibit both the IgE and eosinophil response to helminthic parasites in rodents with a concomitant increase in Th1-lymphocyte response and increased IL-2 and IFN-γ production. Mice genetically engineered to disable the IL-4 gene have no IgE and a markedly reduced eosinophil response to parasite infection. Similarly, therefore, IL-4 antagonists may be expected to be beneficial in asthma.

7.4.5 Immunomodulation

The new emphasis on asthma as a disease caused by a special type of T-cell response to inhaled antigen offers the possibility of a more subtle modulation of the immune response than that offered by non-specific immunosuppressive drugs such as CsA and glucocorticoids. We now have a detailed understanding of the mechanism of the T-cell response to antigen in terms of both the specificity of the response and the intracellular events that follow antigen stimulation. Of particular interest is the observation that T cells can be rendered unresponsive (anergic) if stimulated in a certain manner. This understanding now offers the possibility of intervening to alter an individual's T-cell response to antigen to render the individual either unresponsive or responsive in a non-asthma-inducing fashion. In fact, immunomodulation has been practiced for many years as immunotherapy.

Immunotherapy. This is the technique of administering, usually by subcutaneous injection, increasing amounts of the allergen thought to be causing the symptoms of allergic disease and then maintaining the individual on a fixed dose of allergen, with injections given usually monthly for up to several years, with the aim of desensitizing the individual to that allergen. Initially it was performed with crude extracts, but now purified and semipurified allergens are widely available.

Immunotherapy is still widely practiced in mainland Europe and the USA for both allergic rhinitis, and asthma, but it is rarely used in the UK because of doubts about its safety and efficacy. There is, however, no doubt that immunotherapy can be effective. Immunotherapy has been clearly shown to work in the treatment of seasonal allergic rhinitis (hay fever), using grass pollen allergens, and bee and wasp sting allergy, using allergens derived from venom. There is also good evidence that it can work in atopic asthmatics in whom there is a clearly defined allergic component to a single allergen, usually house dust mite. As might be expected, it is less successful in patients who are atopic to several allergens.

There is little evidence that immunotherapy can cure asthma or allergic disease. The few studies undertaken suggest that symptoms return at some point after stopping treatment, although the optimal length of treatment and the length of remission in successfully treated individuals is uncertain.

Although effective, there is also no doubt that immunotherapy is a potentially hazardous procedure which has a relatively high risk of systemic symptoms due to anaphylaxis, and there have been several well-documented cases of death following allergen injections for immunotherapy. Most of these occurred in asthmatics being desensitized to house dust mite allergen. More problems have been encountered using the purified allergens rather than crude extracts, possibly because they are more potent.

Although the role of immunotherapy in the treatment of asthma remains controversial, the mechanism by which it exerts its effect is potentially informative. Immunotherapy has a number of marked effects on the immune response to allergen, some of which are detailed in *Table 7.8*. Which of these are responsible for its efficacy is uncertain, but the observation that it increases the expression of mRNA for IFN-γ in the skin after allergen challenge suggests it may be promoting a Th1 type of response to allergen at the expense of Th2 cells. In this same study it was observed that immunotherapy reduces mast cell numbers in the skin, suggesting an effect on mast cell growth.

Table 7.8: Immunomodulatory effects of immunotherapy

Type of response	Response observed
(a) *Serum antibody responses*	
IgE	Initial rise and then a fall in specific IgE over several months. Clinical response precedes changes in IgE
IgG	Large increase in allergen-specific IgG, especially IgG4
(b) *Effector cells and mediators*	
Neutrophils	Decrease in serum neutrophil chemotactic activity
Eosinophils	Decreased serum eosinophil chemotactic activity
	Decreased ECP levels in BAL fluid from patients with immunotherapy-treated seasonal birch pollen allergy
	Decreased eosinophil numbers after allergen challenge to nose after immunotherapy in patients with mite-sensitive perennial allergic rhinitis
Mast cells	Decreased numbers of mast cells in skin and nose and mast cell mediators in nasal washings following immunotherapy
T lymphocytes	Suppression of allergen-induced T-lymphocyte proliferation in peripheral blood lymphocytes
	Increased numbers of CD8+ve T cells in skin
	Decreased numbers of CD4+ve cells
	Increased mRNA expression for IL-2 and IFN-γ in some immunotherapy-treated patients after allergen challenge in skin

Recently, the two major epitopes for T cell responsiveness to cat allergen have been isolated and are being marketed as an oligopeptide reagent for immunotherapy (Cat-vax). It will be interesting to see if this very specific antigenic peptide will be effective in modulating the symptoms of people allergic to cat.

Modulation of T-cell responses to allergen. A specific type of T-cell response to inhaled antigen appears increasingly central to the pathogenesis of asthma. As discussed in Chapter 3, antigen is taken up by antigen-presenting cells (APCs), in which it is digested into small peptide fragments. These oligopeptides bind to the groove of HLA class II receptors, which are assembled in the Golgi apparatus and then expressed on the cell surface. The peptide is recognized in association with the HLA receptor by a T-cell receptor specific for that peptide. Any one antigen has a number of peptide regions which are reactive (immunogenic) with T cells. Some immunogenic regions or epitopes are more important (major epitopes) than others (minor epitopes). Attachment of the T-cell receptor to the peptide bound within the class II receptor is not sufficient to cause the T cell to proliferate and produce cytokines. It requires a second signal whose exact nature is uncertain but involves adhesion between the T cell and the APC through one or more accessory receptors on the surface of T cells and their counterstructures on APCs.

Once stimulated, the T cell produces cytokines. As discussed in previous chapters, certain antigens result, in some people, in the T cell producing IL-4 and IL-5, a Th2 type of response, rather than IL-2 and IFN-γ, a Th1 response. IL-4 causes B cells to produce IgE and IL-5 causes increased eosinophil production. This complex series of events allows for intervention at a number of points (*Figure 7.10*).

Although any one oligopeptide can bind a number of HLA class II receptors and any one HLA class II receptor can bind a number of different peptides, there are differing affinities so that one peptide could compete for the binding site of another peptide and so inhibit its ability to provoke an immune response. This has been shown to be effective *in vivo*. Certain strains of mice can be immunized with myelin basic protein in such a way that when they are subsequently re-challenged with myelin-based protein they develop an autoimmune reaction called experimental autoimmune encephalitis (EAE), which is similar in some respects to multiple sclerosis. EAE can also be caused in these sensitized mice by challenge with an oligopeptide taken from a region of myelin basic protein which appears to be immunodominant for this disease. Development of the disease can be blocked by an oligopeptide which has been modified so that it binds more tightly to the class II receptor than the native oligopeptide but is non-stimulatory.

It has been possible to do similar experiments with human T-cell lines and clones specific to house dust mite allergen. A modified peptide derived from influenza virus hemagglutinin was found to be able to inhibit T-cell

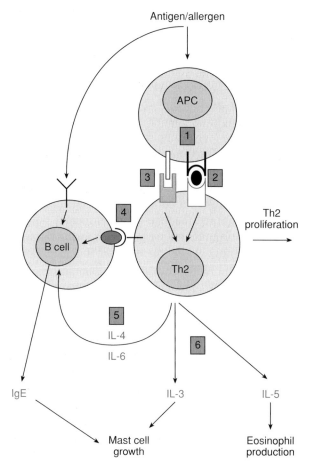

Figure 7.10: Potential sites for immunomodulation. (1) Inhibition of antigen presentation. A number of cells can present antigen in the airways in asthma including B cells, macrophages, dendritic cells and possibly epithelial cells and eosinophils. No strategies have yet been devised to specifically inhibit antigen processing. (2) Designing peptides that bind to the MHC with a higher affinity than allergenic peptides but themselves are non-immunogenic. (3) T-cell activation requires additional signals other than that derived from the antigen receptor. These include signals through accessory receptors on the T cell, such as the adhesion receptors ICAM-1/LFA-1, activation receptors such as CD28 and cytokine signals such as IL-1. Inhibition of these pathways could lead to T-cell anergy or impaired activation. (4 and 5) B cells also require additional signals other than antigen stimulation through their immunoglobulin-like antigen receptor. These include an isotype-specific signal such as IL-4, which causes switching to IgE, a process enhanced by IL-6, and a membrane signal delivered through T-cell adhesion via receptors such as CD40 and CD40 ligand. Antagonists of these cytokines, receptors or their ligands could be effective in preventing IgE production. (6) Antagonists of the end products of Th2 stimulation by allergen may prevent the growth of mast cells and eosinophils.

response to house dust mite allergen from a number of donors *in vitro* by binding more avidly to the HLA class II receptors without provoking a T-cell response in its own right.

Theoretically, a cocktail of peptides could be designed to inhibit the T-cell response to the major epitopes for a number of common allergens as a treatment for asthma, although this is some way off at present. One problem is the number of potential allergens involved and the difficulty in finding peptides which block, but do not themselves cause, an immune response. An alternative strategy is to make the T cells unresponsive. T cells can be rendered unresponsive (anergic) if they are stimulated with antigen in a non-immunogenic form or without the second signal provided by adhesion between APCs and T cells. Similarly, if T-cell clones are stimulated *in vitro* with large amounts of antigenic peptides they fail to proliferate to a second antigen challenge and switch from making IL-4 to making IFN-γ . Whether this feature of T-cell activation can be exploited in some way to change the T-cell pattern of response *in vivo* remains to be seen.

7.4.6 Anti-adhesion therapies

One of the basic properties of the immune response is the ability of leukocytes to migrate out of the blood vessel and into tissue. This process is mediated by several gene families of membrane receptors (see Chapter 3). As well as mediating leukocyte migration, these adhesion receptors are involved in other aspects of the immune system, including acting as accessory signals to allow full T-cell responses to antigen stimulation. Agents that block the action of these receptors have the potential to be powerful anti-inflammatory drugs. Indeed, mAbs directed against some of these receptors have been effective in a number of animal models of human disease (*Table 7.9*).

Table 7.9: Examples of conditions in which anti-adhesion treatment is effective

Adhesion receptor	Condition	Human disease
Leukocyte integrins	Hemorrhagic shock	Shock secondary to blood loss
Leukocyte integrins	Reperfusion injury	Myocardial infarction
		Renal transplantation
Selectins	Reperfusion injury	
ICAM-1	Renal transplantation in baboons	Transplantation
ICAM-1	Allergen-induced eosinophilia and BHR in monkeys	Asthma
VLA-4	Late response to allergen in sheep.	Allergic disease/asthma
	Passive cutaneous anaphylaxis (PCA) reaction in guinea pig	Allergic disease

One set of studies that have excited considerable interest were performed by a group working for Boehringer Ingelheim in the USA. They established a model of asthma in which several inhalation challenges of ascaris antigen were delivered over several days to naturally sensitized monkeys. These monkeys developed an airways eosinophilia and increased bronchial hyperresponsiveness. Anti-ICAM-1 antibodies given either intravenously or by inhalation before the challenges inhibited both the airways eosinophilia and the increased BHR. Whether this was a direct effect on eosinophils or due to an effect on T cells or monocytes was not clear. Unlike glucocorticoids, if the anti-ICAM-1 was given after challenge no effect was seen, suggesting that this antibody could block migration of cells into the lung but unlike the steroids could not reverse the process once it had started.

Anti-adhesion treatment has now reached the stage of clinical trials in renal transplantation. However, there are a number of problems to be overcome before it is likely to be used routinely in the treatment of asthma. Mouse mAbs may sensitize the individual and are therefore unsuitable for chronic treatment. Humanized mAbs may be more acceptable. Blocking adhesion is potentially immunosuppressive, as seen in leukocyte adhesion deficiency. Ideally, specific adhesion pathways will be blocked in specific diseases so that this problem is avoided, but the evidence that this is going to be possible is still limited. The receptor pair VLA-4/VCAM-1 is not expressed by neutrophils, and there is some evidence from animal models that these receptors are important in eosinophil migration. They may therefore be useful target receptors for anti-adhesion therapy in asthma.

7.4.7 Cytokine therapy

Th2 cells are inhibited by IFN-γ. It might therefore be expected that IFN-γ would be effective in the treatment of asthma. Both IFN-γ and the related IFN-α are available for clinical use, and have been used in hypereosinophilic syndrome, in which both drugs are promising; in hyper-IgE syndrome, in which patients have a very high serum IgE, skin rashes and immunosuppression, and in which early reports are also promising; and in atopic dermatitis, for which IFN-γ appears to be effective. No trials of IFN-γ in asthma have been reported, but it can be safely given by inhalation and its effects in asthma are awaited with interest.

Further reading

General

Barnes, P.J. (Ed.) (1992) *New Drugs for Asthma*. IBC Technical Services, UK.

Buckle, D.R. and Smith, H. (Eds) (1984) *Development of Anti-Asthma Drugs*. Butterworths, London.

Glucocorticoids

Brown, P.H., Teelucksash, S., Matusiewicz, S.P., Greening, A.P., Crompton, G.K. and Edwards, C.R.W. (1991) Cutaneous vasoconstrictor response to glucocorticoids in asthma. *Lancet*, **337**, 576–580.

Corrigan, C.J., Brown, P.H., Barnes, N.C., Szefler, S.J., Tsai, J.J., Frew, A.J. and Kay, A.B. (1991) Glucocorticoid resistance in chronic asthma. *Am. Rev. Respir. Dis.*, **144**, 1016–1025.

Corticosteroids: their biological mechanisms and application to the treatment of asthma. *Am. Rev. Respir. Dis.*, **141**, Supplement 2, part 2.

Dutoit, J.I., Salome, C.M. and Woolcock, A.J. (1987) Inhaled corticosteroids reduce the severity of bronchial hyperresponsiveness in asthma but oral theophylline does not. *Am. Rev. Respir. Dis.*, **136**, 1174–1178.

Flower, R.J. (1988) Lipocortin and the mechanism of action of the glucocorticoids. *Br. J. Pharmacol.*, **94**, 987–1015.

Gustafsson, J.A., Carlstedt-Duke, J., Poellinger, L. *et al.* (1987) Biochemistry, molecular biology and physiology of the glucocorticoid receptor. *Endocrine Rev.*, **8**, 185–234.

Hollenberg, S.M., Weinberger, C., Ohg, E.S., Cerelli, G., Oro, A., Levo, R., Thompson, E.B., Rosenfeld, M.G. and Evans, R.M. (1985) Primary structure and expression of a functional human glucocorticoid receptor cDNA. *Nature*, **318**, 635–641.

Laitinen, L.A., Laitinen, A. and Haahtela, T. (1992) A comparative study of the effects of an inhaled corticosteroid, budesonide, and a β_2-agonist, terbutaline, on airway inflammation in newly diagnosed asthma: a randomized, double blind, parallel group controlled trial. *J. Allergy Clin. Immunol.*, **90**, 32–42.

Munck, A., Mendel, D.B., Smith, L.J. and Orti, E. (1990) Glucocorticoid receptors and actions. *Am. Rev. Respir. Dis.*, **141** (Suppl. 2), S2–S10.

Taylor, I.K. and Shaw, R.J. (1993) The mechanism of action of corticosteroids in asthma. *Respir. Med.*, **87**, 261.

Wilkinson, J.R.W., Crea, A.E.G., Clark, T.J.H. and Lee, T.H. (1989) Identification and characterization of a monocyte-derived neutrophil activating factor in corticosteroid-resistant bronchial asthma. *J. Clin. Invest.*, **84**, 1930–1941.

β_2-Agonists

Anon. (1990) β2 agonists in asthma: relief, prevention, morbidity. *Lancet*, **336**, 1411–1412.

Inman, W.H.W. and Adelstein, A.M. (1969) Rise and fall of asthma mortality in England and Wales in relation to use of pressurized aerosols. *Lancet*, **2**, 279–285.

Jackson, R.T., Beaglehole, R., Rea, H.H. and Sutherland, D.C. (1982) Mortality from asthma: a new epidemic in New Zealand. *Br. Med. J.*, **285**, 771–774.

Jenne, J.W. and Tashkin, D.P. (1993) Beta-adrenergic agonists. in *Bronchial Asthma. Mechanisms and Therapeutics*, 3rd Edn (E.B. Weiss and M. Stein, Eds). Little Brown & Co., Boston, p. 700.

Immunosuppressive agents

Alexander, A.G., Barnes, N.C. and Kay, A.B. (1992) Trial of cyclosporin A in corticosteroid-dependent chronic severe asthma. *Lancet,* **339,** 324–328.

Calderon, E., Lockey, R.F., Bukantz, S.C., Coffey, R.G. and Ledford, D.K. (1992) Is there a role for cyclosporine in asthma? *J. Allergy Clin. Immunology.,* **89,** 629.

Mullarkey, M.F. (1993) Potent anti-inflammatory agents. in *Bronchial Asthma, Mechanisms and Therapeutics,* 3rd Edn (E.B. Weiss and M. Stein, Eds). Little Brown & Co., Boston.

Mullarkey, M.F., Blumenstein, B.A., Andrade, W.P., Bailey, G.A., Olason, I. and Wetzel, C.E. (1988) Methotrexate in the treatment of corticosteroid dependent asthma: a double blind cross-over study. *New Engl. J. Med.,* **318,** 603–607.

Schreiber, S.L. (1992) Immunophilin-sensitive protein phosphatase action in cell signalling pathways. *Cell,* **70,** 365–368.

Shiner, R.J., Nunn, A.J., Fan Chung, K. and Geddes, D.M. (1990) Randomized, double blind, placebo-controlled trial of methotrexate in steroid dependent asthma. *Lancet,* **336,** 137–140.

Sigal, N.H. and Dumont, F.J. (1992) Cyclosporin A, FK-506 and rapamycin: pharmacologic probes of lymphocyte signal transduction. *Annu. Rev. Immunol.,* **10,** 519–560.

Bronchodilators

Giembycz, M.A. (1992) Could isoenzyme-selective phosphodiesterase inhibitors render bronchodilator therapy redundant in the treatment of bronchial asthma? *Biochem. Pharmacol.,* **43,** 2041–2051.

Giembycz, M.A. and Dent, G. (1992) Prospects for selective cyclic nucleotide phosphodiesterase inhibitors in the treatment of bronchial asthma. *Clin. Exp. Allergy,* **22,** 337–344.

Small, R.C., Berry, J.L., Burka, J.F., Cook, S.J., Foster, R.W., Green, K.A. and Murray, M.A. (1992) Potassium channel activators and bronchial asthma. *Clin. Exp. Allergy,* **22,** 11–18.

Mediator antagonists

Alexander, A. and Barnes, N. (1993) New drugs in asthma, in *Asthma and Rhinitis* (S. Holgate and W. Bussey, Eds). Blackwell Scientific Publications, Oxford, Ch. 104, in press.

Kopf, M., Le Gros, G., Bachmann, M., Lamers, M.C., Bluethmann, H. and Kohler, G. (1993) Disruption of the murine IL-4 gene blocks the Th2 cytokine response. *Nature,* **362,** 245–248.

Sher, A., Coffman, R.L., Hieny, S. and Cheever, A.W. (1990) Ablation of eosinophil and IgE responses with anti-IL-5 or anti-IL-4 antibodies fails to affect immunity against *Schistosoma mansoni* in the mouse. *J. Immunol.,* **145,** 3911–3916.

Immunomodulation

Chapman, M.D. (1991) Use of non stimulatory peptides: a new strategy for immunotherapy? *J. Allergy Clin. Immunol.*, **88**, 300–302.

O'Hehir, R.E. and Lamb, J.R. (1992) Strategies for modulating immunoglobulin E synthesis. *Clin. Exp. Allergy*, **22**, 7–10.

O'Hehir, R.E., Yssel, H., Verma, S., de Vries, J.E., Spits, H. and Lamb, J.R. (1991) Clonal analysis of differential lymphokine production in peptide and superantigen-induced T cell anergy. *Int. Immunol.*, **3**, 819–826.

Varney, V.A., Gaga, M., Few, A.J., Aber, V., Kay, A.B. and Durham, S.R. (1991) Usefulness of immunotherapy in patients with severe summer hayfever uncontrolled by anti-allergic drugs. *Br. Med. J.*, **302**, 265–269.

Anti-adhesion therapies

Harlan, J.M. and Liu, E. (Eds) (1992) *Adhesion: Its Role in Inflammatory Diseases*. W.H. Freeman & Co., New York.

Wegner, C.D., Gundel, R.H., Reilly, P., Haynes, N., Letts, G. and Rothlen, R. (1990) Intercellular adhesion molecule-1 (ICAM-1) in the pathogenesis of asthma. *Science*, **247**, 456–459.

Zimmerman, G.A., Prescott, S.M. and McIntyre, T. (1992) Endothelial interactions with granulocytes: tethering and signaling molecule. *Immunol. Today*, **13**, 93–100.

Chapter 8

Conclusions and summary

Asthma is one of the most common and universal of diseases, affecting all ages, at all times and in all places. It is a disorder characterized by variable airways obstruction caused by a combination of constriction of bronchial smooth muscle, mucus plugging, and thickening of the bronchial wall due to smooth muscle hypertrophy and mucosal edema. These pathological abnormalities are in turn caused by inflammation of the airways, characterized pathologically by an eosinophilic infiltration of the bronchial wall and activation of a specific type of lymphocyte subset. The inflammatory process leads to the airways being unusually sensitive (hyperresponsive) to non-specific irritants such as smoke and noxious fumes.

A major cause of the airways inflammation is likely to be a T cell-mediated response to inhaled antigens, of which allergens such as house dust mite and animal furs as well as occupational allergens/antigens play an important role. For many asthmatics, viral infections both trigger and exacerbate asthma. The link between viral infections and the immune response in asthma is still poorly understood.

Clinically, asthma can vary from an occasional cough with slight wheeze to a life-threatening and chronically incapacitating disease. It is often hard to envisage these clinical phenotypes as being part of the same disease. Indeed, there is still a debate as to whether asthma is one disease or whether the various clinical patterns represent separate diseases with different etiologies. The evidence either way is not conclusive. However, where they have been established, the pathological changes in all patterns of asthma are very similar, suggesting a common pathogenesis.

Considerable progress has been made in the last 10 years in understanding the cellular and molecular basis of asthma, particularly the nature of the inflammatory response. This understanding has been greatly aided by parallel developments in other chronic inflammatory diseases and by dramatic advances in our understanding of basic mechanisms in human biology, particularly the basis of specific immunity, the events leading to leukocyte migration into tissue, the mediators involved in the inflammatory process, and the intracellular signaling pathways that result in mediator release and effector cell function. These in turn have opened up new avenues for treatment which will undoubtedly lead to new types of drugs for asthma to complement the effective and safe medications that have found their places in clinical practice over the last two decades.

It is sometimes said that basic research has a limited impact on the management of a disease, but asthma is a good example of a condition whose clinical management has been directly influenced by research. Although it has been known for almost a century that asthma is characterized by airway inflammation, both treatment and ideas about pathogenesis had tended to focus on the physiology and pharmacology of bronchial smooth muscle spasm, with the emphasis on bronchodilation. It was not until the last 10 years that, as a result of fiber-optic bronchoscopy studies pioneered by investigators in France, it became obvious that airway inflammation was at the root of even the mildest forms of the disease. As a result there has been an increasing emphasis on the need to use anti-inflammatory drugs at an early stage to prevent airway inflammation.

We know a great deal about the nature of the inflammatory response in asthma. Less clear are the factors that influence the very varied response to that inflammatory process, particularly in the area of bronchial hyperresponsiveness. Why does one individual with evidence of eosinophilic inflammation of the airways have few symptoms, whereas another with a similar degree of airways inflammation has catastrophic disease? Similarly, the relationship between atopy and asthma remains uncertain. Between 30 and 50% of the population is atopic and yet only perhaps a third will suffer from allergic symptoms and many less from asthma. Why do some atopic individuals have rhinitis or eczema but no asthma, and vice versa? Why does asthma in any one individual suddenly start, wax and wane, and then often disappear, without any obvious change in environmental circumstances.

Even in terms of the inflammatory response many questions remain. What are the factors leading to resolution or non-resolution of inflammation after exposure to a trigger such as inhaled allergen? Is the eosinophil really a pivotal cell? Perhaps most importantly, what is it that makes a person respond to certain antigens with a Th2-type response? If we knew we might be able to turn it into a Th1 type of response and possibly cure the disease.

Many questions remain, but we live in exciting times and the answers may not be far off.

Appendix A. Glossary

Acquired (adaptive) immunity: the part of the immune system that responds in a specific manner to foreign antigen.

Adenylate cyclase: enzyme that catalyzes the synthesis of cyclic AMP from ATP. A key component of one of the second messenger pathways.

Adhesion receptors: a large and heterogenous group of membrane receptors that control a large number of cellular functions including cell motility, embryogenesis and wound healing.

Airflow obstruction: a condition of the airways in which the flow of air in and out of the lungs is impaired by narrowing or blockage of the bronchi.

Alleles: two or more alternative forms of a gene at a particular chromosomal location (locus).

Allergen: a foreign, non-parasite, antigen that can cause a specific IgE response in some individuals.

Antigen: an agent, usually a foreign protein, that causes a specific immune response.

Asthma: a disease characterized by variable airflow obstruction, bronchial hyperresponsiveness and an eosinophilic inflammation of the airways.

Atopic: a person who has generated specific IgE against one or more allergens as defined by a positive skin prick test or a positive *in vitro* test for specific IgE (e.g. RAST test).

Atopic disease: diseases related to a specific IgE response to allergens. These include atopic (extrinsic) asthma, atopic dermatitis (eczema) and allergic rhinitis.

Autocrine: a mediator that acts on the cell by which it was produced.

B lymphocyte: cell that makes immunoglobulin.

Bronchi: airways below the trachea which have cartilage in their walls.

Bronchial hyperresponsiveness: increased sensitivity of the airways to noxious stimuli.

Bronchiole: airway without cartilage.

CD: a number given by an international workshop to a membrane structure recognized by two or more monoclonal antibodies. Usually defines a glycoprotein membrane receptor.

Chemokines: a family of chemotactic cytokines.

Chromosome: structure in the nucleus on which genes are located. Humans have 22 paired autosomal chromosomes, and one X and Y chromosome (male) or two X chromosomes (female).

Cyclic AMP: a second messenger that activates protein kinase A and is linked to the adenylate cyclase signal transduction pathway.

Cytokines: group name for a complex and heterogenous mixture of peptide mediators released by a number of cell types that modulate cell function in a variety of ways. They often have a role in controlling cell growth and differentiation.

Eicosanoids: inflammatory mediators derived from arachidonic acid.

Epitope: region of a protein recognized by the antigen recognition structures of either immunoglobulin or the T cell antigen receptor.

Extrinsic (atopic) asthma: asthmatics who have specific IgE to common allergens.

FcεRI: high affinity receptor that binds IgE. Expressed by mast cells and basophils.

FcεRII: lower affinity receptor that binds IgE. Expressed by B cells, macrophages and platelets.

Fiber-optic bronchoscopy: technique to examine directly the major airways using a flexible fiber-optic scope.

Forced expiratory volume in one second (FEV$_1$): measurement of lung function that measures how much air is expelled in 1 sec. The FEV$_1$ is low in asthma.

Gene: segment of DNA that encodes for an RNA and/or polypeptide.

Gene therapy: therapeutic intervention by altering the genetic make up of a tissue or individual. At the moment this usually involves inserting a normal gene into the organ where a defective gene is expressed.

Genotype: (a) the genetic constitution of an individual; (b) the types of alleles found at a locus in an individual.

Glucocorticoids: a group of 21-carbon corticosteroids produced in the adrenal cortex. Glucocorticoids have marked anti-inflammatory activity, and synthetic glucocorticoids are one of the most effective preventative therapies for asthma.

G protein: a protein that binds GTP and is linked to a range of membrane receptors with a common seven transmembrane structure. Engagement of the receptor results in a change in the structure of the G protein, which triggers a number of second messenger events. G protein activation is an early step in many signal transduction pathways.

Haplotype: description of the types of alleles found at linked loci on a single chromosome.

Haptens: low molecular weight chemicals which on their own are non-antigenic but which become antigenic when they bind to other proteins in the blood, such as albumin.

Helminthic parasites: metazoan parasites (worms). They generally provoke an eosinophilia and production of IgE.

Human leukocyte antigens (HLA): receptors (class 1 and class 2) expressed on the surface of a variety of cells which bind antigenic peptide fragments in order to present them to the T cell antigen receptor, so resulting in a specific (i.e. directed only against that antigen) immune response.

Immunoglobulin gene superfamily: large gene family coding for membrane receptors involved in immune recognition.

Immunophilin: family of intracellular proteins that bind immunosuppressants related to cyclosporine.

Innate immunity: the part of the immune system which is not dependent on recognition of specific antigens for its function. Includes the complement system, phagocytosis, anti-bacterial components of saliva.

Integrins: a large family of adhesion receptors characterized by a two chain heterodimeric structure.

Interleukins: a subclass of cytokines that were initially defined as regulating lymphocyte proliferation and activation, although this is not always the case, e.g. IL-8, which is a chemoattractant.

Intrinsic asthma: asthmatics who are non-atopic.

Isotype: class of immunoglobulin.

Leukotrienes: class of lipid mediators including the sulfidopeptide leukotrienes (LTC_4, LTD_4 and LTE_4), previously called slow relaxing substance of anaphylaxis (SRS-a), and LTB_4 derived from arachidonic acid by the action of the enzyme 5-lipoxygenase.

Ligand: the structure which binds to a receptor. Often called a counter-structure or counter-receptor.

Lymphoblast: activated lymphocyte.

Major histocompatability complex (MHC): the region of chromosome 6 (in humans) where the genes for the human leukocyte antigens (HLA) are located.

Memory T cells: T lymphocytes that have been stimulated by antigen through their antigen receptor.

Messenger (m)RNA: strand of nucleic acid transcribed from a gene which passes into the cytoplasm and is translated into protein on ribosomes.

Monoclonal antibodies: antibodies which recognize the same antigenic epitope.

Mutations: alterations in the nucleotide sequence of a DNA molecule.

Naive T cells: T lymphocytes that have not encountered antigen.

Non-specific triggers: irritant stimuli that provoke an asthma attack in people who already have asthma.

Peak expiratory flow (PF/PEF): measures the maximum flow rate at which air is expelled (in $l\ sec^{-1}$). It is reduced in asthma and is the most convenient way to monitor the severity of asthma objectively.

Phenotype: the appearance or other characteristics of an organism.

Phosphatidylinositol: a phospholipid involved in another class of second messenger pathways which results in calcium influx and protein kinase C activation.

Plasma cell: antigen-stimulated, Ig-producing B cell.

Polymorphism: a variable DNA sequence, one that can exist in a number of different, although related forms.

Prostaglandins and thromboxanes: lipid mediators derived from arachidonic acid by the action of the enzyme cyclo-oxygenase.

Protein kinase: enzyme that catalyzes the phophorylation of proteins on serine, threonine or tyrosine residues.

Provocational concentration causing a 20% fall in FEV₁ (Pc20): investigation to measure the degree of bronchial responsiveness.

Reverse genetics (positional cloning): process by which the gene responsible for a given phenotype is identified by locating its position on the chromosome by linkage to other known regions of DNA.

Selectins: a structurally related family of adhesion receptors characterized by an N terminal lectin domain.

Signal transduction: process by which the signal resulting from a ligand binding to its receptor (usually a membrane receptor) is transmitted into the cell and the early events subsequent to that signal being delivered.

Skin prick test: test to identify specific IgE, in which the skin is lightly scratched with a needle through a drop of allergen extract. A positive reaction is denoted by a wheal and flare. The size of the wheal is taken as the size of the response.

Specific triggers: stimuli that interact with the immune system to provoke an inflammatory response in the airways leading to asthma. Usually refers to allergens or viral infections.

T lymphocyte: cells involved in cell-mediated immunity and B lymphocyte help.

Th2/Th1: T lymphocyte subsets with characteristic profiles of cytokine secretion.

Transcription: the synthesis of an RNA copy of a gene.

Transgenic mice: mice genetically engineered by insertion of a specially designed gene into the germline, which results in either inhibition or overproduction of the protein encoded by the gene.

Translation: the process of making a peptide (protein) chain from a strand of mRNA.

Wheal and flare: reaction in which an edematous papule (wheal) appears on the skin surrounded by an erythematous reaction (flare). In the context of the skin prick test it is due primarily to the release of vasoactive mediators, such as histamine, from skin mast cells.

Index